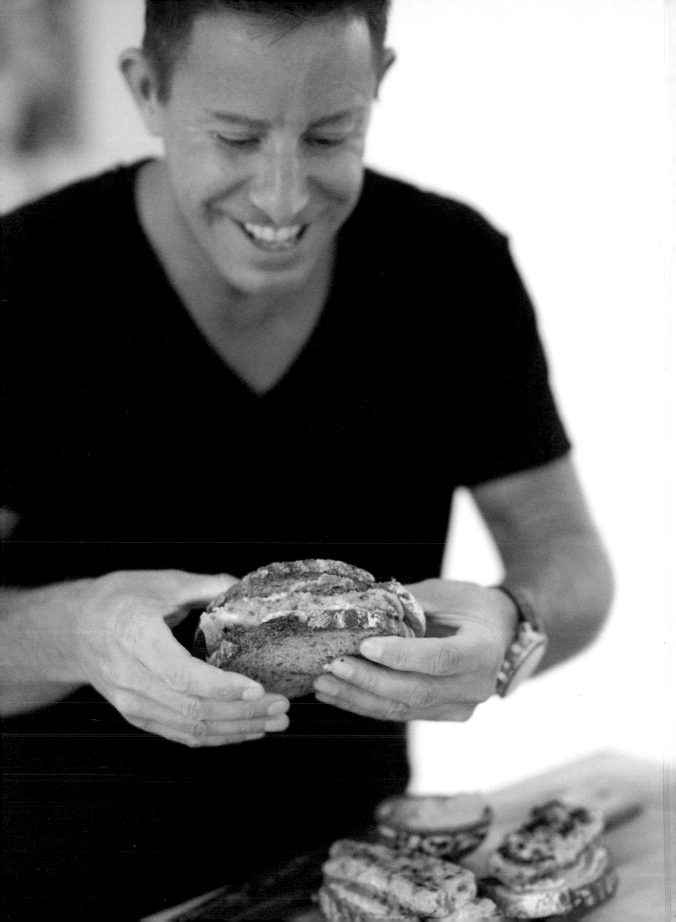

JASON VALE

SUPER *fast* FOOD

No Chef Required!

Thank You!

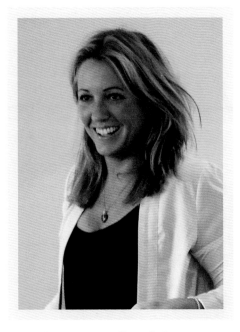

My Beautiful KATIE...

This picture of my lovely Katie shouldn't be on this page, to be fair it should be on the front cover! To say Katie has 'helped' with this book would be perhaps the biggest understatement ever made. Not only has Katie massively helped to produce some of the finest *'Super fast Food'* ever created, but she was also the person responsible for making virtually all of the recipes for the photography in this book. There was no 'food stylist' or big crew. The vast majority of the photographs were the result of Katie simply making the dishes, dressing the set and Alex snapping them with his magic photography eye. Katie is a stickler for detail and wanted to make sure every single recipe was unique and hit all the *Super fast Food* buttons. Together, I hope you'll agree once you start to tuck in, myself and Katie have produced not only a beautifully looking book, but a book with recipes which are uncomplicated, that anyone can make, and which hit all the nutritional buttons without being 'boring'. Katie also painstakingly went through and triple checked every page before going to print, a task which took a couple of 12 hour days!

So Katie, I would like to say a genuine, massive and very public **THANK YOU!** Thank you particularly for caring so much and for helping to make my first whole food recipe book one to be super proud of. Thank you for being the person you are daily. Thank you for being a bright light in many people's lives, none more so than mine. Thank you for just being your extremely unique, caring, giving, beautiful self. ***THANK YOU! THANK YOU! THANK YOU!*** And I'll see you tonight for a ***Super fast Food*** dinner :)

PS: When's 'Deliciously Katie' coming out?

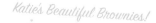
Katie's Beautiful Brownies!

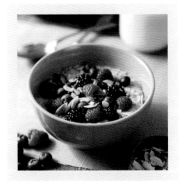
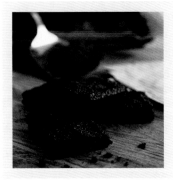
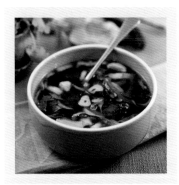

The photo king – it's **ALEX LEITH** people!

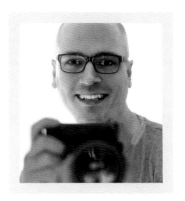

This is Alex, someone whom I have had the great privilege of knowing and working with over the past decade. Alex, together with his lovely wife Charlie, are a couple of life's rare ones. The best way to describe them is 'beautiful people creating beautiful work'. Alex has filmed almost everything I have ever done, videos, apps, etc, and this dynamic duo were also the people behind the groundbreaking documentary, Super Juice Me! I could wax lyrical for pages about just how brilliant he (they) are, but unfortunately I don't have the space here. So all I will say here is: Alex, **THANK YOU!** Thank you for being so flexible. Thank you for never saying no. Thank you for always making time. Thank you for the sheer quality and caring that goes into everything you do and ***THANK YOU, THANK YOU, THANK YOU*** not only for the stunning photos in this book, but also for a great book jacket and intro. You, my man, are da bomb!

Let's give it up people, for the one and only **ANDREA WELLS**!

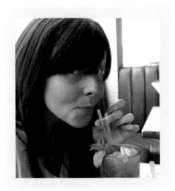

This is Andrea, my P.A. and general all-round wonderful egg. Andrea is again one of life's unusual treasures. I have had the honour of knowing and working with Andrea for a quite a few years now and to say she wears many hats in the company – other than 'P.A.' – would be an understatement! Once again it would be extremely easy to wax lyrical about this truly amazing woman for many pages, but space is our enemy! So, Andrea, **THANK YOU!** Thank you for being there whenever I need you. Thank you for always going above and beyond the call of duty. Thank you for caring so much for others. Thank you simply for being the person you are and, in terms of this book, ***THANK YOU, THANK YOU, THANK YOU*** for reading, re-reading and re-reading again the many pages of this book to make sure that what goes out isn't littered with mistakes. It was a long journey, but BOOM! ***Super fast Food*** is here in the flesh and look, you're in it! :)

And finally... let's give it up for **DAVID & OLIVIA**!

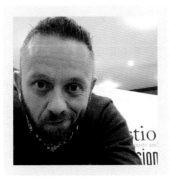

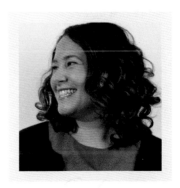

The wonderful David is the person who did the vast majority of the typesetting and layout for this book and the equally beautiful Olivia, who works over at Print Data Solutions, has been the one responsible for managing all things printing. David and Olivia, what can I say? We got there! That, I am sure you'll agree David, was a longer journey than any of us envisaged. So, I would like to say **THANK YOU!** Thank you for adapting. Thank you for listening. Thank you for your design prowess and ***THANK YOU*** guys for making sure this bad boy got printed on time!

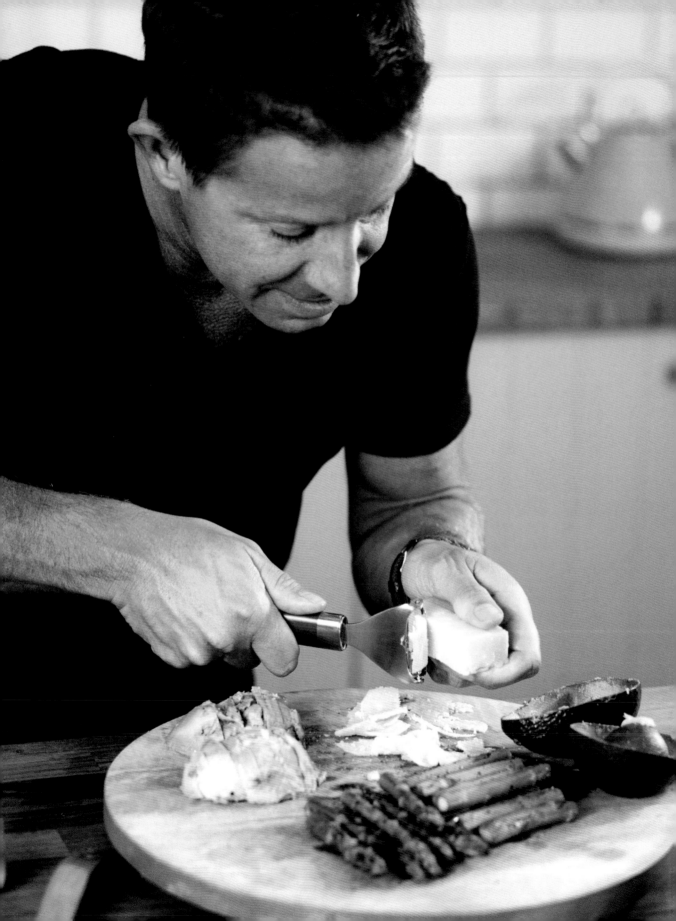

CONTENTS

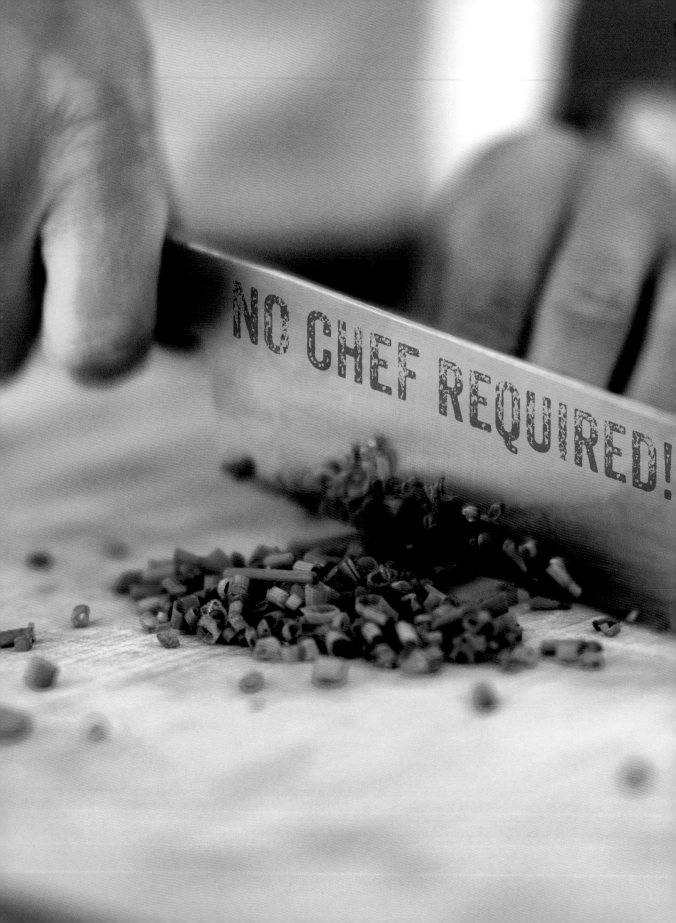

"YES CHEF!
NO CHEF!"

If you ever find yourself in a professional working kitchen in a top restaurant, *'YES CHEF!'* is something you'll hear hollered a great deal. However, find yourself in *my* kitchen when I'm making dinner and **'CHEF'** is not a word you'll ever hear.

To be clear from the start, *I'm not a chef.* I can't chop an onion into perfect little cubes in four seconds flat, whilst moving my knife at a hundred miles-an-hour, nor can I make the perfect tarte tatin – but the chances are neither can you. That's why all of the recipes in this book are *non-chef* and *non-pretentious* proof; meaning all are made with unpretentious, uncomplicated and recognizable ingredients. All of the recipes have been carefully constructed with the **'NO CHEF REQUIRED!'** mantra throughout. In fact, if you get a chance to watch any of the recipe videos on the **Super fast Food** app, you'll soon realize just how *un-chef-like* I am and just how easy these recipes are to make.

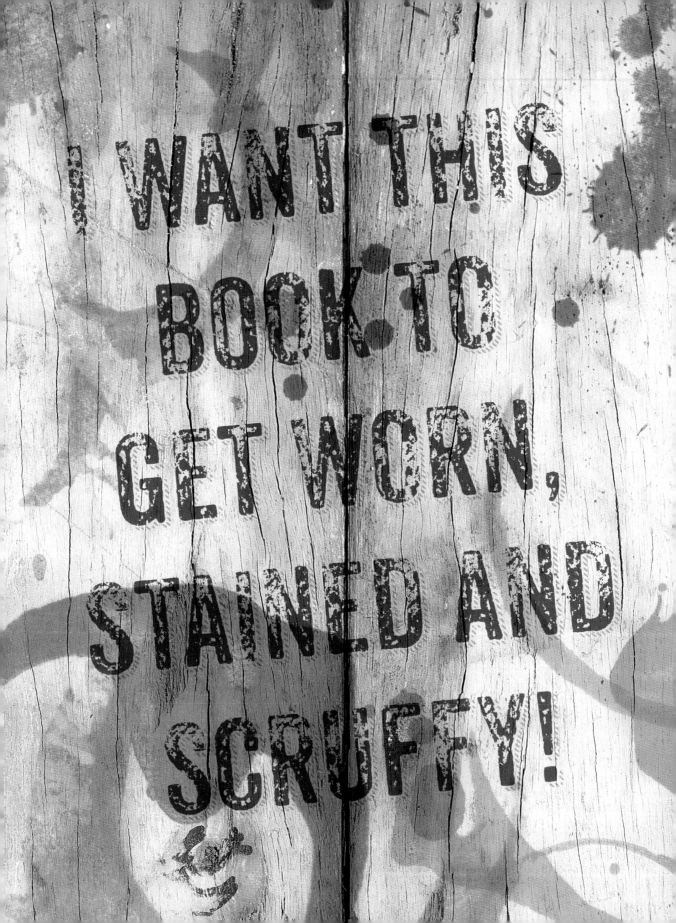

HERE'S TO A RECIPE BOOK YOU MIGHT ACTUALLY USE!

It's worth knowing from the off, that in the UK we buy more recipe books than any other country in Europe, yet at the same time we buy twice as many take-a-ways. We also love a good cookery show, with over 434 hours being beamed into UK homes each and every week. (Yes, that's **434 HOURS**!) The hard truth is, that the vast majority of cookbooks are used as decorative features on kitchen shelves, rather than what they were intended for, and most cookery shows are used as 'food voyeurism' and 'entertainment' rather than for genuine inspiration or to *actually* make what you've just seen.

I know this first hand as I have a beautiful array of Jamie, Nigella and Gordon books gracing my shelves, all looking beautiful and as brand new as the day someone bought them for me! All, no doubt, wonderful books with amazing recipes, but I don't know because I've never actually made any of them! Equally I have watched many, many cookery shows with amazing

recipes, but have yet to get off the sofa to actually make any of them. From the gastronomical genius of Heston Blumenthal to the incredibly charismatic Mr. Gordon Ramsay cooking up a storm on shows like *Cook Along with Gordon*, I'm as mesmerized as the next person.

The problem is I don't ever actually get off my arse and do what the programme makers intend, i.e. to cook along with Gordon or join Jamie for two hours and actually *make* one of his '30 Minute' Meals. (That was a joke Jamie… well, joke-*ish*!) Nope! Instead I'll make something quick and easy; with ingredients I know, using as few pans as possible and in the shortest possible time. I'll then sit in front of the TV with my **Super fast Food** meal, turn on *Master Chef* and spend the next hour trying to decipher the utterly pretentious descriptions given to the so called 'every day' recipes they're about to prepare. FYI, 'roasted fillet of Australian Kobe beef nestled in a Kent garden puree, temptingly accompanied by a succulent spinach and onion compote, to die for triple-cooked Maris Piper chips and Indonesian long pepper sauce,' is basically beef, peas, spinach, chips and gravy to me and you (do you really need to cook chips three times?) Then you have Nigella! I think it's fair to say most watch Nigella not so much because they wish to replicate the food she's making, but more for the added 'sultry factor' she brings to the kitchen table!

Yes, food voyeurism is rife and like me, most people are extremely good at *watching* cooking shows and *looking* at the pictures of recipe books! A recent survey showed that the average person makes just four recipes from a cookbook. Meaning Jamie, Nigella and Gordon don't take pride of place in our kitchens because we need quick access for our daily use, but rather as the unspoken message to visitors of, *'Hey, look at my cook books, aren't they lovely and yes, in case you're wondering, I take home-cooking very seriously'* — even though in reality cobwebs may be holding the pages together!

SUPER FOOD
SUPER FAST
SUPER EASY

The aim of *this* book is to buck that trend and I honestly hope it does. I want this book to get worn, stained, sticky and scruffy. I want the pages stuck together – not with cobwebs because its been left to rot on the shelf, but with the bits of food that got splattered over the book whilst you were making the delicious recipes within. I want this book to reignite your cooking fire and show you just how frighteningly easy it can be to eat well.

I want this book to become part of your daily life, the *go-to* book of choice for taste, flavor and optimum nutrition. I also want this to be the book you immediately go to after you have finished one of my Juice Challenges in order to keep you on the healthy road to success. I want to show you that delicious and extremely nutritious

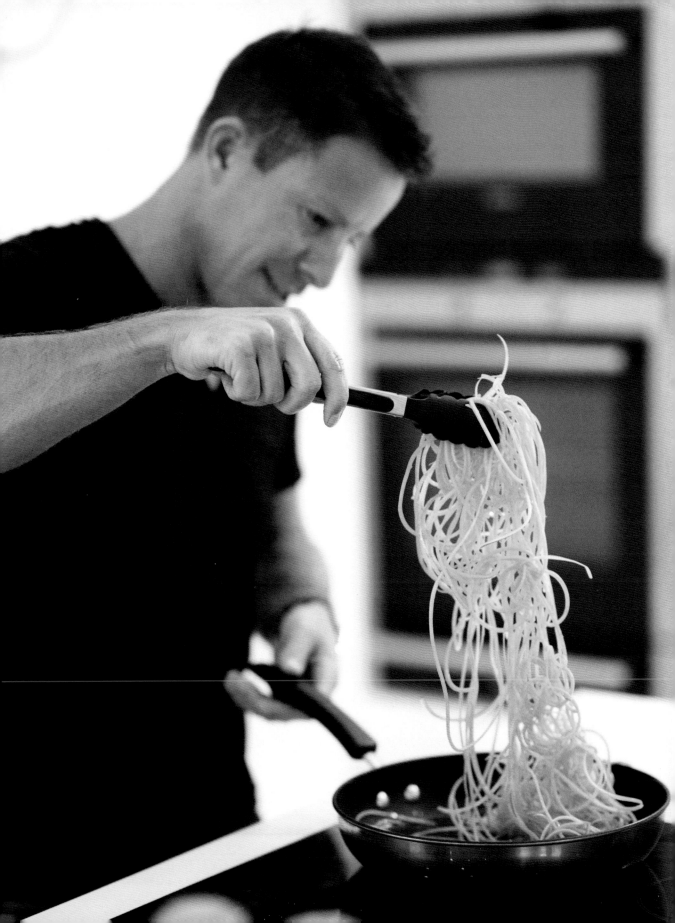

meals can indeed be made in super fast time, with normal ingredients by even the clumsiest of 'would-be' chefs.

This, I feel, is one of the most inviting aspects about the recipes in this book. You won't find any random or obscure ingredients that can only be found in an Amazonian rainforest (or a trendy shop in Notting Hill — one and the same really!) I have only used ingredients that can be found in most major supermarkets. I have also made sure that those ingredients can be 'crossed over' to help minimize waste and make your **Super fast Food** cooking life as cost effective and convenient as possible. This means that once you have **The Staples** (page 22) tucked away in your larder, you'll have the core foundation so all you will need to get are the fresh ingredients to make the recipes contained within this book.

I almost called this book *UNCOMPLICATED* or *UNPRETENTIOUS*. Both good titles, I feel, and both words that sum up quite nicely what this book represents. In the end though, I opted for **Super fast Food** as that's essentially what you'll find — superfood meals that can be prepared in super fast time! You may think that it's going to be extremely hard to find, superfoods in major supermarkets, but first we need to ask:

WHAT IS A 'SUPERFOOD' ANYWAY?

As far as I'm concerned the definition of a superfood is pretty straightforward. It is any food that was designed by nature for human consumption and one which hasn't been denatured or bastardized beyond all recognition. A superfood is simply any food that adheres to the original Hippocrates mantra of, '**Let Food Be Thy Medicine & Medicine Be Thy Food**'. A true superfood is one that has the ability to both feed and heal, rather than slowly destroy and damage.

If you go back to the '40s, '50s, '60s etc. there was no such term as superfood. Why? Because back then it was just food! I honestly believe the very term 'superfood' has only come about since the invention, if you will, of *non*-superfoods. Clearly, if you live in a developing country and are genuinely starving, then I believe it could be argued that *all* food is a superfood, including things like refined sugar and fats. However, when you are lucky enough to have a choice over what you eat (and I am guessing the vast majority of people reading this book will fall into this category) then not all food is the same and some foods are indeed 'super' by comparison.

In the wild, *all* animals **only** consume superfoods; or simply *food* as they know it. All food consumed in the wild is eaten in its natural, 'live' state; animals don't cook their food — ever! A squirrel, for example, would never describe the nuts it eats as a superfood; to the squirrel it's just food. However, if all the other nuts were covered in fat, salt and sugar; heavily processed and no longer contained the genuine nutrition of a natural nut, then the natural, unprocessed nut could be defined as 'super'. This is because it will have nutritional and healing properties that the heavily processed nuts no longer have.

I agree that the term *superfood* sounds ridiculous and probably feels completely made up in order to sell you some berries that can only be found in the far reaches of the planet (I have no doubt some use it for that purpose) but the reason why things like goji berries, acai berries, blueberries, broccoli, ginger, spinach, turmeric, cucumber, mango and so on are often referred to as superfoods is because, compared to the heavily processed crap most people are eating and drinking, they are!

It's like the first time I saw Fairtrade bananas. All it did was draw my attention to the fact that all the rest were in some way *unfair*. There shouldn't have to be Fairtrade bananas any more than there should be superfoods, but in a world of unfair bananas and heavily processed foods, these terms have unfortunately become necessary.

You can now get most superfoods in all major supermarkets, but then I'd argue you always could. **Avocados, broccoli, rocket, watercress, tomatoes, cucumber, ginger, cabbage, berries, bananas, eggs, lean proteins, seeds, nuts,** and **grains** are all ***superfoods***, but because they are so common and 'non exotic' they no longer seem to get the superfood status they deserve. I am aware I keep referring to supermarkets and this might give the impression that I no longer support local farms where possible, however, I only refer to the fact you can get all the ingredients in supermarkets so you know all of the recipes are accessible to everyone – not just the ones living near Borough Market! The good news is that as well as the mainstream superfoods (fruits, vegetables, lean proteins, seeds, nuts etc., etc.) you can now get most of the new kids on the superfood block such as acai, goji, quinoa, coconut oil etc. almost anywhere too. Once you have **The Staples** (page 22) in your cupboard, you are set up beautifully for your new *Super fast Food* lifestyle.

What I am trying to hammer home is that regular, everyday, natural foods are superfoods. In fact, it was these very superfoods I turned to in my hour of need. It was these superfoods I juiced like they were going out of fashion, blended like my life depended on them and ate 'till the cows came home'. It

was these true superfoods that helped to completely transform my own personal health which is why these apparent non-exotic 'regular' foods will always have a big fat 'super' before them in my book.

For me, the ultimate superfood is the humble avocado. It is the only food, which it is said, you can live on exclusively (you'll have no friends clearly) but avocados contain everything the human body needs. I believe in avocados so much that I credit them for changing my life. They are my 'butter' of choice, you can eat them straight from their own 'bowl' as the perfect snack and they turn any regular fresh juice into a truly satisfying superfood blend. I believe it was the good fats, along with the amino acids, vitamins, minerals, enzymes and organic water contained within these amazing fruits that helped to clear me of my aliments… of which I had many!

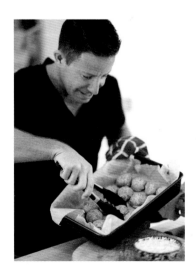
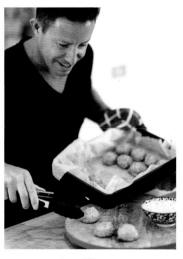
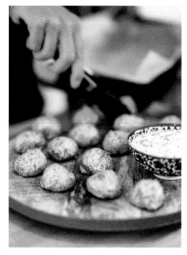

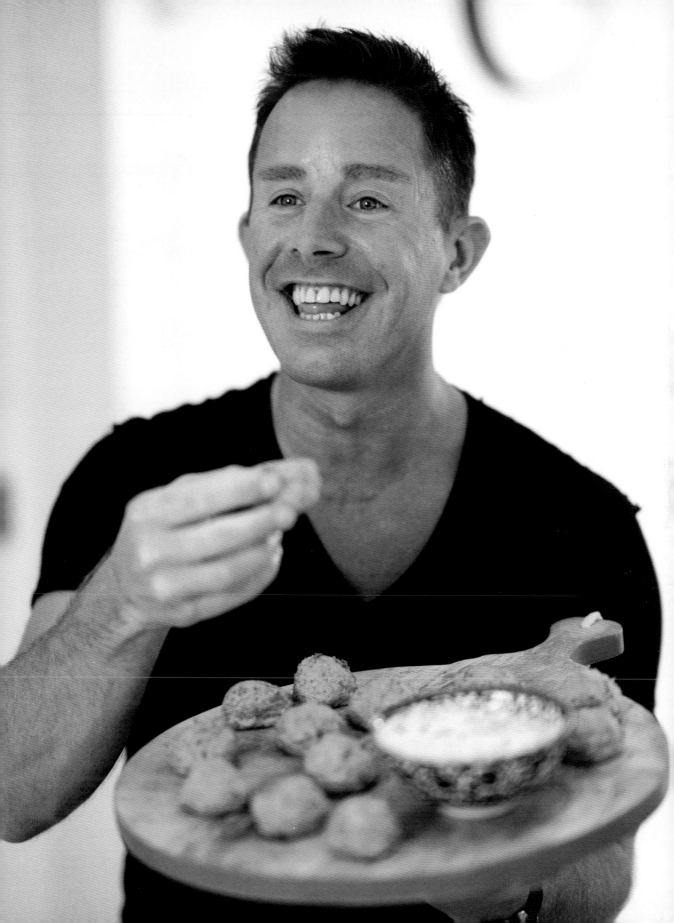

NO MORE MR. FLAKEY, WHEEZY FAT BOY!

To give you just an extremely quick look at what has led me to write so passionately about this subject for over 15 years, here's my story in brief. I was covered from head to toe in a skin condition called psoriasis (over 90% of my body was affected). I had extremely severe asthma (using both the blue and brown steroid inhalers up to 14 times a day). I also suffered with bad eczema and hay fever. On top of this I used to smoke 2–3 packets of cigarettes a day, drank alcohol to oblivion, consumed other drugs (I was a Peckham boy) and was also a fat little camper. I never ate anything natural, and I paid the price heavily for it.

I made a decision to change my diet completely, so out went the cigarettes, the alcohol and all processed foods; and in came the fresh vegetable juices, beautiful salads, good grains and lean proteins. Once I did this, what happened to me can only be described as miraculous. My asthma vanished, my psoriasis went, no more eczema and **no more Mr. Fat Guy**! Surely the only description you can give to the foods which transformed my health to such an extent is 'super'?

I wish to be clear, this isn't a 'I'll fix all your health issues' book – it's a healthy recipe book. I am not a doctor, nor am I suggesting that just because *I* experienced these changes with the exclusive inclusion of superfoods, that you, or indeed anyone else reading this book, will have the same success (there, disclaimer done!) However, I think we all intuitively know that by cutting out the rubbish and adding in the good stuff, our health (and waistline) is going to improve to some extent!

IT'S ALL ABOUT LOW H.I. EATING
NOT PERFECTION!

In case you are wondering, my life doesn't consist of living on a diet of nothing but superfoods and fresh juice, trust me, I'll never be that person who rushes home to tuck into some raw broccoli for fun! Life, and 'being human', is clearly about balance.

You can *try* to play the food and drink 24/7 perfection game, but ultimately you'll lose. You'll lose a great deal of your life for starters! I have seen this time and time again where people become so obsessed with every single little thing they put in their body that it ultimately creates even more hardship than when they suffered at the hands of junk food! **They end up so focused on trying to extend their life that they miss having a life in the process.** *(I know – I was there!)* What they have done is not *remove* a food problem, but simply *move* a food problem.

If you play the perfection game you also lose a few more things, usually some of your friends (who wants to hear you banging on about gluten-free and raw food all the time?) and often you'll also lose *the very will to live*!

***Balance* is key**, for we are human after all, but it needs to be the right balance or we pay a pretty hefty price. Go too far in either direction on the food front and you tend to be screwed. This is why, most of the time, I adhere to what I describe as 'low H.I eating' and why all the recipes in this book adhere to these

criteria. Low H.I stands for low 'Human Intervention'. In other words, no matter what the food or drink, I ask myself 'how much has a human interfered with it?' The more it has been interfered with, the worse it tends to be. Simple! No more looking at every ingredient on a label, just ask yourself 'is it low H.I?' *(Although the fact that it even has a label is usually a sign that it isn't!)* An orange picked directly from a tree for example is *no* H.I but something like a heavily processed refined sugar-and fat-laced muffin is *high* H.I

We need to understand that only wild animals eat nothing but no H.I foods. To do the same, we'd also have to live in the wild and have skills like Bear Grylls just to be able to survive. Luckily we don't need to eat no H.I in order to be slim and healthy. The body can deal with a certain amount of just about *anything* and still stay healthy. We have an inbuilt filter system, which is the reason why, despite smoking heavily, drinking heavily and eating crap from morning till night, I'm still here! But, if I had carried on I honestly feel I *wouldn't* be here today, as the body can only deal with a certain amount (and not the bucket-loads that I was pouring in).

What this illustrates is that, if you have a cappuccino, some processed cheese or a cheeky 'one' with your friends, for example, you won't get ill or die! This bodes well for this book as not every dish has exclusive superfood ingredients. It's all about getting the right balance. Clearly not many would describe halloumi cheese as a superfood but equally it's not high fructose corn syrup either! One thing you can guarantee is that each recipe is as low H.I and as 'superfood friendly' as possible, without compromising on interesting and moreish textures and flavors and without it not feeling like 'real' food.

THERE'S MORE TO LIFE THAN
QUINOA & CAULIFLOWER RICE!

This was also another title I toyed with for this book, as that's how I genuinely feel. Yes, you will find some quinoa and cauliflower rice in this book, they are genuine superfoods after all and low H.I, but you'll also find *actual* rice as well as *actual* cheese (I know I'm a maverick, what can I tell you!) This is why my favorite section in this book is **The Classics** (page 175). Here you'll find healthy versions of things like Thai curry, lasagna, pizza, fish 'n' chips, chilli, shepherd's pie, spaghetti Bolognese, bangers 'n' mash and even a burger – you know, things you actually recognize and dishes the whole family can enjoy together without people thinking you're some kind of health freak!

IT'S NOT ALL ABOUT THE JUICE!

Clearly, given I have written over ten books on the subject, I could never write a full recipe book without mentioning freshly extracted juice. Not only am I mentioning it here, but I have also included some wonderful blend options for breakfast. If you have read any of my juice books, you'll know just how important a role I feel fresh juice needs to play in the average persons' diet. I also feel, like servicing your car, it is vital

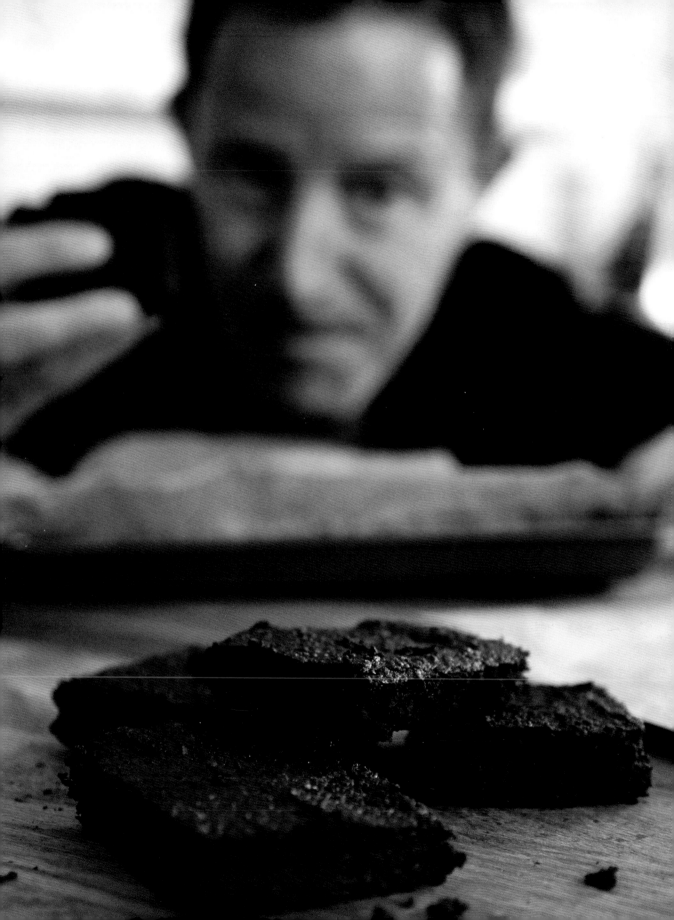

to put your body in for a regular service too. After over fifteen years of writing about health, I have yet to see anything which is more effective for rapid, healthy weight loss (and good health in general) than a well thought through *juice-only* plan.

I only mention this because I have no idea how you came across this particular book and you may be suffering from some health or weight issues. If that's you, then I cannot emphasize strongly enough what kicking off your superfood lifestyle with a pure juice plan first, can do for you. Not only does the average person drop at least 7lbs in seven days, but also something incredible tends to happen to your cravings. You start out by thinking all you'll want at the end of the seven days is the stuff that got you into health and weight trouble in the first place. And you finish literally craving

low H.I superfoods and drinks. I have seen this happen to tens of thousands of people over the years and most describe it as a 'reset'. I reset myself and put my system in for a full-on 'juice service' four times a year without fail. I also live on nothing but freshly extracted juice for two days a week as part of my **5:2 Juice Diet** principles.

This type of lifestyle may well not float your boat or fit into your world. Even the thought of living on nothing but juice for a week has the average person reaching for the donuts before you can say, 'juice me up!' But if you've never experienced one and need that final nudge to try a juice challenge on for size, please make sure you watch the groundbreaking documentary *Super Juice Me!* first. It's **100% FREE to watch** on YouTube or at **www.superjuiceme.com**.

SUPER FOOD ME!

If a pure *juice-only* challenge isn't quite for you, then you'll be pleased to know I have included a couple of **Super food Me!** *7-Day Plans* in this book (one veggie and one pesci). These superfood plans still get incredible results and will still help you to achieve the most important aspect of long-term change, by 'resetting' your mind and biochemistry. The body and mind tends to crave what it has on a regular basis. Eat well *most* of the time and you'll be naturally drawn to *want* to eat well most of the time. Eat crap *most* of the time and you'll be drawn to *want* to eat crap most of the time. This is why, in an ideal world, I recommend kicking off with one of my juice plans first.

Clearly if you are a healthy bunny already, then you may well not need a juice plan, or even the **Super food Me!** *7-Day Plans* at all, you'll simply dip in and out of this book making recipes that complement your already healthy lifestyle.

You may have just completed one of my *juice-only* plans which lead you to this book. If that's you, then again I would highly recommend picking one of the two **Super food Me!** *7-Day Plans* as they are the perfect follow-on. And I will reiterate, if you are in a bad way on the health and weight front and you really can't do *juice-only*, then you'll find either of the plans will suit you beautifully and help to kick things off in a wonderful way. **Super food Me! 7-Day Plans** *(pages 30-33)*

APPY MEAL!

The **Super fast Food** app was released way before this book, and went straight in at No. 1 (even knocking Jamie Oliver off the top spot... something I don't talk about often, as you can imagine ☺). It's a great companion to the book, especially if you wish to **Design Your Own Plan**. You can select any breakfast, lunch, dinner, side and sweet; assign them to a day and create your own 1, 2, 3, 4, 5, 6 or 7-day meal plan. It will even go a step further and generate a shopping list for your own plan.

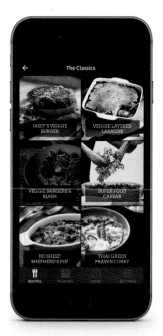

I made a decision that the app will never have any in-app purchases, and future updates will always be free. I am aware this seems like an ad, but if you love the recipes in the book and would like the opportunity to create your own plan *(and get to watch me make the recipes)* then the app does the job nicely.

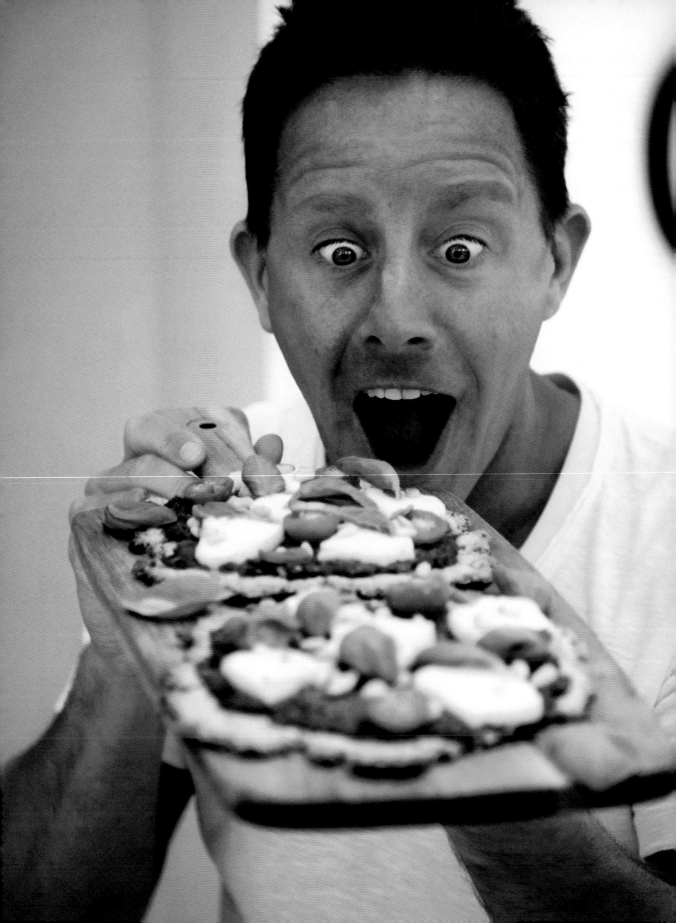

MOMENTUM IS KEY...
SO LET'S GET CRACKING!

If you are serious about making *Super fast Food* a lifestyle and something you intend to live by the vast majority of the time, then I have suggested four simple steps to help get you off the ground. Before I lay those out, I would like to say a big **'THANK YOU'** for picking up the book, and I honestly hope it helps to make a genuine difference to your world. I love hearing from people, especially if they've had a major transformation having followed one of my plans. So if you find you have had success on the health or weight loss front and you don't mind dropping me a line, I'd love to hear from you:

✉ testimonials@juicemaster.com 🐦 @juicemaster
ⓕ facebook.com/juicemasterltd ⊙ @jasonvale
▶ youtube.com/juicemaster Ⓖ +juicemaster

At the time of writing this book I am also building another health retreat in the Algarve in Portugal (where you might find a few of these recipes make a showing!) If you are ever there, we may even get to 'do lunch'.

Whether our paths cross or not, I wish you and yours the very best of health.

Big Love,
Jason

"IF YOU DON'T LOOK AFTER YOUR BODY YOU'LL HAVE NOWHERE TO LIVE!"

YOUR
4 STEPS TO
SUPER
FAST
FOOD
SUCCESS

STEP 1. GET THE STAPLES

The Staples are ingredients that keep for a long time and are used in most recipes time and time again – so get **The Staples** (page 22)

STEP 2. PICK A SUPER FOOD ME! 7-DAY PLAN

There are two to choose from: one with fish (pesci option) and one without (veggie option). You can, of course, design your own plan based on your preferences.

STEP 3. GO SHOPPING & SET A START DATE

There are three ways to get your shopping list:

1. *They are on pages 34-35 of this book.*
2. *They are free to download at www.juicemaster.com*
3. *They are on the app.*

Clearly if you are designing your own plan, you'll have to work out the shopping for yourself; or the *Super fast Food* app can do this for you. It's key to set a date and most tend to choose a Monday. This means Sunday is your shopping day and most people have more time on a Sunday than on most other days, which gives plenty of time to grab **The Staples** and the other ingredients needed for your plan. However, don't be surprised if when you get home with all of your amazing superfoods, that after you have packed them away, you then pick up the phone to get a take-a-way! This is because we are human and that's what we do before we start any healthy eating plan. What this tends to do is help the cause, as half way through the junk food stuffed crust pizza, we are hating ourselves so much that we can't wait get started.

STEP 4. DON'T STRIVE FOR PERFECTION!

As I mentioned at the start, I'm not a chef and the chances are neither are you. Please do not strive to make each meal 'perfect'. As long as it tastes great and you've used the ingredients suggested in the way I have suggested, then tuck in and enjoy.

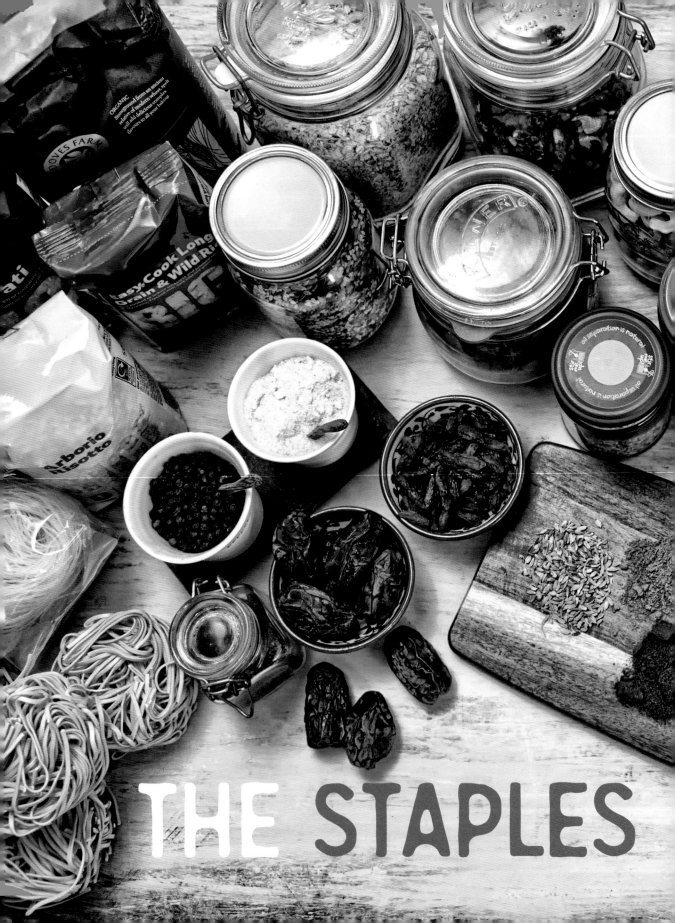

THE STAPLES

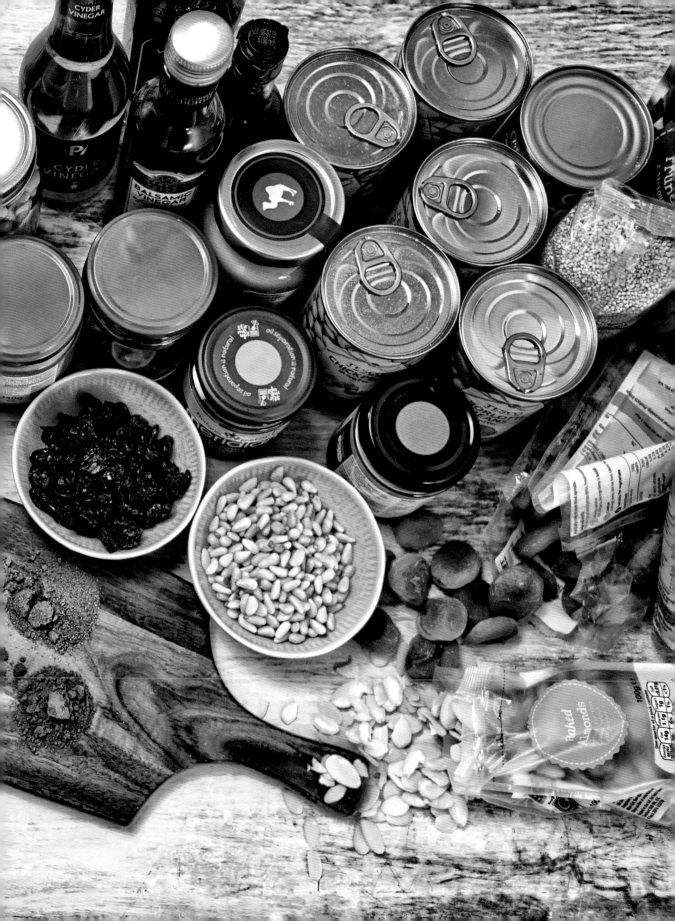

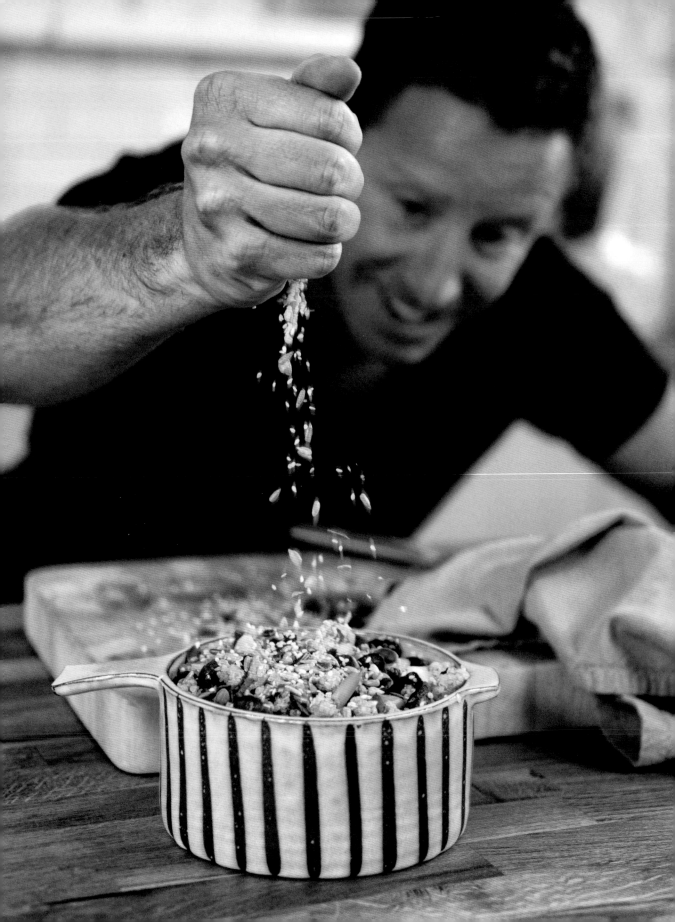

PREPARE YOURSELF FOR SUCCESS!

In today's busy world, it's all too easy to talk yourself out of cooking a good healthy meal, especially after a long hard day at work and a tiresome journey home.

Your food intentions may have been good and pure at the start of the day but before you know where you are, the dreaded C.B.A ('Can't Be Arsed') Syndrome has reared its ugly head; the phone is in your hand and you're ordering a not so healthy take-a-way. The key here is to ensure that rustling up a *Super fast Food* meal is almost as easy as 'ordering in'. I can assure you that in the long run, nothing will put a nail in your *Super fast Food* coffin quicker than not having the necessary staple ingredients in your cupboard and/or freezer. If you have to go out and get every single tiny ingredient each time you want to make a recipe from this book, the chances are you just won't bother. Picking up one or two fresh ingredients isn't an issue, but it's the having to think about whether you have **The Staples** to go with them that can easily put a halt to healthy proceedings.

This is why I highly recommend stocking up on the following key ingredients as they are used in many of the recipes. Then all you have to think about buying on the day are the main headline 'fresh acts' in the dish, such as vegetables, fruits, fresh herbs, fish or cheese etc. Many of the ingredients you will probably already have in your cupboard anyway, so this shouldn't be a big investment and it will mean you are armed and ready to make pretty much any of the recipes whenever you fancy.

What you will notice, as promised in the intro, is that all of **The Staples** are regular, simple, recognizable ingredients that can be found in any major supermarket. So before you embark on your *Super fast Food* journey, take just one trip to your local store, pop **The Staples** in your basket and I promise you'll be a happy camper that you did.

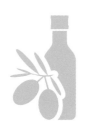

OILS & VINEGARS

Olive Oil *(preferably cold-pressed)*   Apple Cider Vinegar
Coconut Oil   Sesame Seed Oil
Balsamic Vinegar

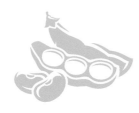

CANNED BEANS & PEAS

Borlotti Beans   Black Eyed Beans
Kidney Beans   Butter Beans
Chickpeas   Garden Peas *(frozen are fine)*

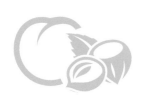

DRIED FRUITS, NUTS & SEEDS

Apricots   Ground Almonds
Raisins   Cashews
Sultanas   Hazelnuts
Dates *(Medjool are well   Pine Nuts
    worth the investment)*   Pecans
Goji berries   Pumpkin Seeds
Dried Cranberries   Mixed Seeds
Prunes   Poppy Seeds
Almond Nut Butter   Sunflower Seeds
Almonds
Flaked Almonds

SEASONING, SPICES & HERBS

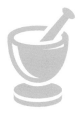

Black Pepper

Himalayan Rock Salt

Cinnamon

Nutmeg

Ground Turmeric

Ground Cumin

Cayenne Pepper

Fennel Seeds

GRAINS

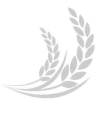

Quinoa

Couscous

Wild Rice Combo

Basmati Rice

Risotto Rice

CONDIMENTS & OTHERS

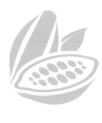

Tahini

Soy Sauce *(or gluten free
alternatives such as Tamari
or Braggs Liquid Aminos)*

Dijon Mustard

Honey *(good quality or
vegan alternative such
as date/rice syrup)*

Sun-Dried Tomatoes

Capers

Coconut Milk

Coconut Water

Vegetable Stock Cubes

Cacao or Cocoa

Self Raising Flour *(gluten-free)*

Oats

Egg Noodles
(or gluten-free alternative)

Rice Noodles

Rye Bread

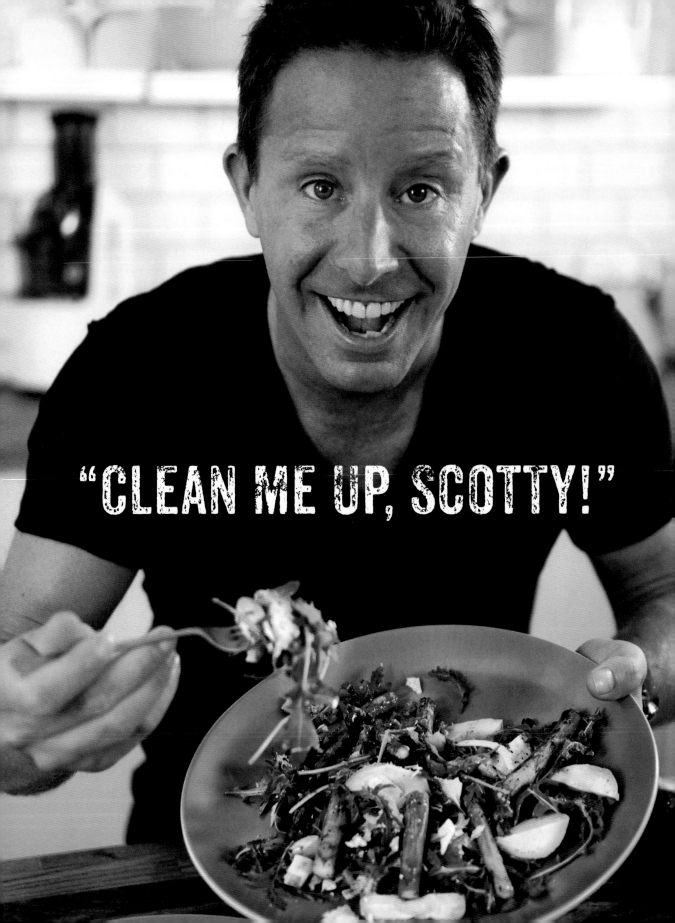

"CLEAN ME UP, SCOTTY!"

SUPER
food
ME!

Your 7-Day Cleanup!

DAY 4

DAY 5

DAY 6

DAY 7

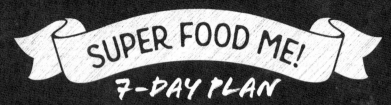

SUPER FOOD ME!

7-DAY PLAN

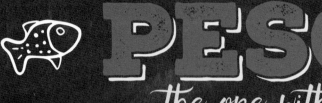 

PESCI
the one with fish

DAY 1

DAY 2

DAY 3

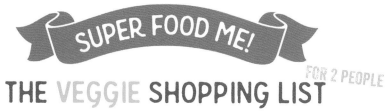

THE VEGGIE SHOPPING LIST

FOR 2 PEOPLE

BAKERY

Gluten-Free Buns	2
Rye Bread (or gluten-free alternative)	2 slices

CANNED GOODS

Red Kidney Beans	500g
Butter Beans / Lima Beans	100g

CEREALS

Rolled Oats	225g

CONDIMENTS, OILS & SEASONINGS

Coconut Oil	45 ml
Himalayan Rock Salt	
Black Pepper (ground)	
Extra Virgin Olive Oil	300ml
Apple Cider Vinegar	30ml
Vegetable Stock Cube	1 cube
Balsamic Vinegar	40ml
Sesame Oil	45ml
Dijon Mustard	7ml

DAIRY

Parmesan	110g
Crème Fraîche	80ml
Halloumi	450g
Natural Yogurt (or vegan alternative)	45g
Eggs (organic, free-range)	12
Butter	25g
(unsalted organic, or vegan alternative)	

DELICATESSEN

Olives (pitted)	70g
Sun-Dried Tomatoes	175g

DRINKS

Coconut Water	400ml
Raw Almond Milk	1 litre
Half-Fat Coconut Milk	600ml

DRY GOODS

Rice Noodles	300g

Couscous	150g
Risotto Rice	200g
Basmati Rice	150g

FREEZER

Ice	

FRESH HERBS

Basil	100g
Fennel	½ bulb
Mint	175g
Dill	20g
Garlic	14 cloves
Raw Ginger	100g
Thyme	10g
Coriander	10g

DRIED FRUIT, NUTS & SEEDS

Dried Apricots	6
Raisins	20g
Dried Cranberries	20g
Flaked Almonds	45g
Pine Nuts	50g
Fennel Seeds	15g
Mixed Seeds	25g
(sunflower, pepita, sesame, chia, etc.)	
Almonds	150g
Sunflower Seeds	10g
Pumpkin Seeds	10g
Cashew Nuts	100g

PRODUCE

Pears	2
Cucumbers	½
Avocados	4½
Courgettes	2½
Celery	2 stalks
Carrots	2
Parsnips	3
Red Bell Peppers	4
Yellow Bell Peppers	3
Red Onions	4½
Medjool Dates	8
Bananas	2
Spinach Leaves	250g
Spring Onions	3

Oranges	2
Lemons (unwaxed)	1¾
Fresh Garden Peas (or frozen)	275g
Wild Rocket	40g
Apples (Golden Delicious or Gala)	2
Sweet Potatoes	4
Raw Beetroots	1 bulb
Beef Tomatoes	2
Goji Berries	20g
Blackberries	80g
Blueberries	40g
Raspberries	40g
Mange Tout	120g
Baby Leaf Spinach	100g
Edamame Beans	60g
Butternut Squash (medium)	½
Red Chillis (medium)	5
Limes (unwaxed)	2
Cauliflower	1
Mixed Berries	100g
(blueberries, blackberries, raspberries, strawberries or seasonal)	
Tomatoes	14
Romaine Lettuce (small)	1
Cherry Tomatoes (on the vine if possible)	30
Portabello Mushrooms	2
Sugar Snap Peas	60g
Broccoli	150g
Kale	50g

SPICES

Ground Turmeric	1.5g
Ground Cumin	2.5g
Ground Red / Cayenne Pepper	2.5g

SPREADS

Almond Butter	45g
Honey (or natural vegan sweetener)	25g
Tahini Paste	30g

SUPPLEMENTS

Spirulina	10g

MISC

Wooden Skewers	6

GENERATE DAY-BY-DAY SHOPPING LISTS ON THE APP

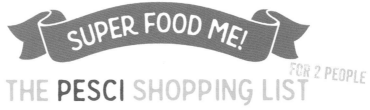

THE **PESCI** SHOPPING LIST

FOR 2 PEOPLE

BAKERY

Gluten-Free Buns	2
Rye Bread *(or gluten-free alternative)*	2 slices

CANNED GOODS

Red Kidney Beans	250g
Butter Beans / Lima Beans	100g

CEREALS

Rolled Oats	225g

CONDIMENTS, OILS & SEASONINGS

Coconut Oil	75 ml
Himalayan Rock Salt	
Black Pepper *(ground)*	
Soy Sauce	30ml
Extra Virgin Olive Oil	325ml
Stock Cube	1 cube
Balsamic Vinegar	70ml
Sesame Oil	45ml

DAIRY

Parmesan	150g
Crème Fraîche	80ml
Halloumi	450g
Natural Yogurt *(or vegan alternative)*	45g
Eggs *(organic, free-range)*	12
Butter	25g
(unsalted organic, or vegan alternative)	

DELICATESSEN

Olives *(pitted)*	70g
Sun-Dried Tomatoes	175g

DRINKS

Coconut Water	400ml
Raw Almond Milk	1 litre
Half-Fat Coconut Milk	600ml

DRY GOODS

Egg Noodles	150g
Couscous	150g
Risotto Rice	200g
Basmati Rice	150g

FREEZER

Ice

FRESH HERBS

Basil	130g
Fennel	½ bulb
Mint	150g
Dill	10g
Garlic	15 cloves
Raw Ginger	100g
Thyme	10g
Coriander	40g

FISH

Salmon Fillets	4
Monkfish	300g
Fresh King Prawns *(peeled, uncooked)*	200g

DRIED FRUIT, NUTS & SEEDS

Dried Apricots	6
Raisins	20g
Dried Cranberries	20g
Flaked Almonds	45g
Pine Nuts	50g
Fennel Seeds	15g
Mixed Seeds	25g
(sunflower, pepita, sesame, chia, etc.)	
Almonds	150g
Sunflower Seeds	10g
Pumpkin Seeds	10g
Cashew Nuts	100g

PRODUCE

Pears	2
Cucumbers	½
Avocados	4½
Courgettes *(medium)*	1½
Celery	2 stalks
Red Chillis *(medium)*	4
Carrots *(medium)*	1
Parsnips *(large)*	2
Red Bell Peppers	2½
Yellow Bell Peppers	2
Red Onions	3½
Medjool Dates	8
Bananas	2
Spinach Leaves	250g
Spring Onions	5

Oranges *(large)*	2
Lemons *(unwaxed)*	4
Fresh Garden Peas *(or frozen)*	175g
Wild Rocket	40g
Apples *(Golden Delicious or Gala)*	2
Sweet Potatoes	6
Raw Beetroots	1 bulb
Beef Tomatoes *(large)*	2
Goji Berries	20g
Blackberries	80g
Blueberries	40g
Raspberries	40g
Mange Tout	200g
Baby Leaf Spinach	100g
Edamame Beans	60g
Pak Choi	1
Limes *(unwaxed)*	1
Cauliflower	1
Mixed Berries	100g
(blueberries, blackberries, raspberries, strawberries or seasonal)	
Tomatoes	10
Romaine Lettuce *(small)*	1
Cherry Tomatoes *(on the vine if possible)*	30
Portabello Mushrooms	2
Sugar Snap Peas	60g
Broccoli	150g
Kale	50g
Asparagus	150g

SPICES

Ground Turmeric	1.5g
Ground Cumin	2.5g
Ground Red / Cayenne Pepper	2.5g

SPREADS

Almond Butter	45g
Honey *(or natural vegan sweetener)*	30g
Tahini Paste	30g

SUPPLEMENTS

Spirulina	10g

MISC

Wooden Skewers	6

DOWNLOAD **THE SHOPPING LISTS FROM** WWW.JUICEMASTER.COM

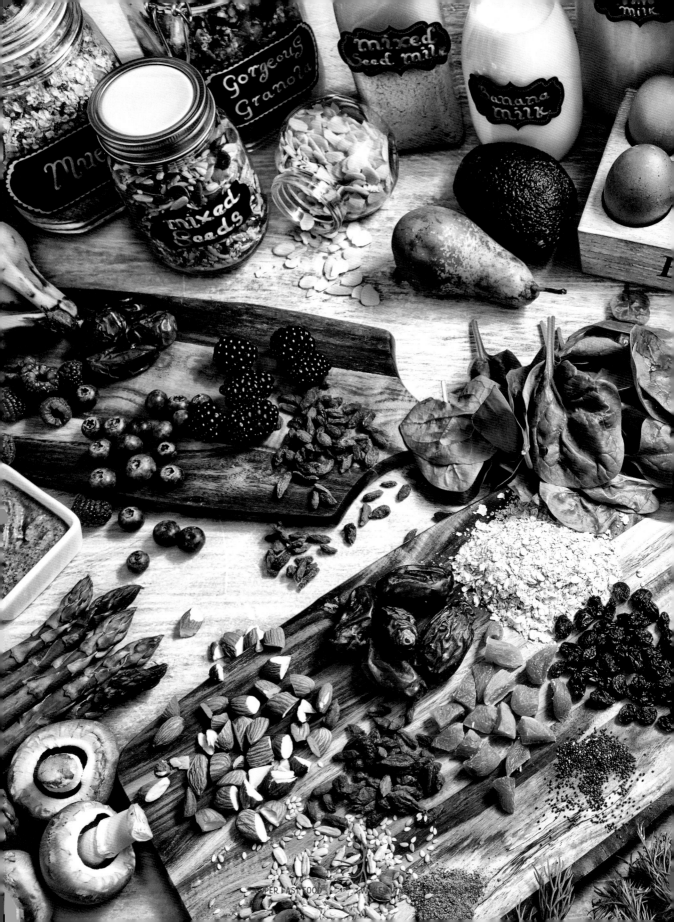

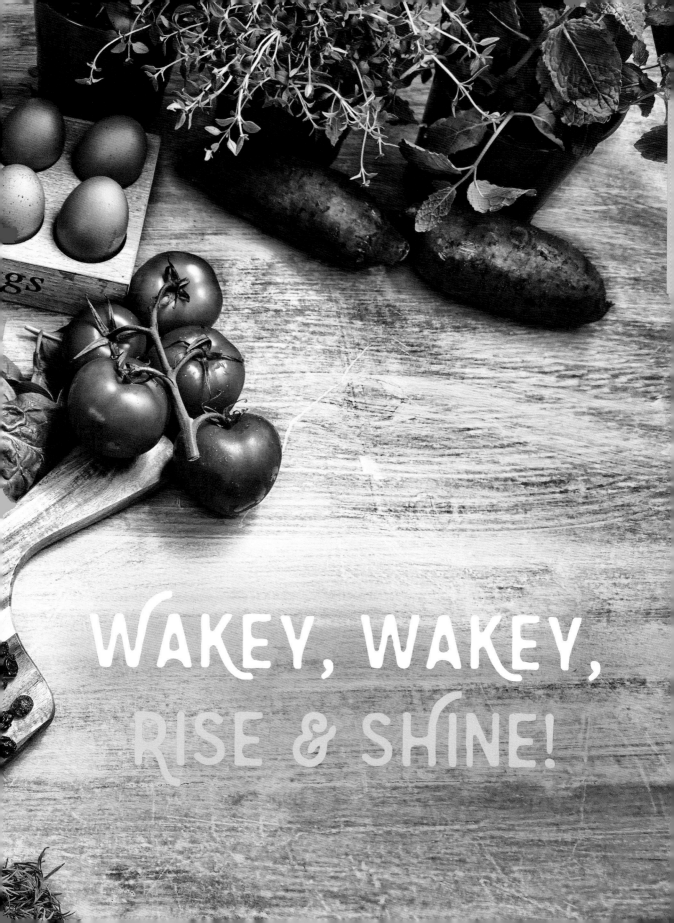

WAKEY, WAKEY,
RISE & SHINE!

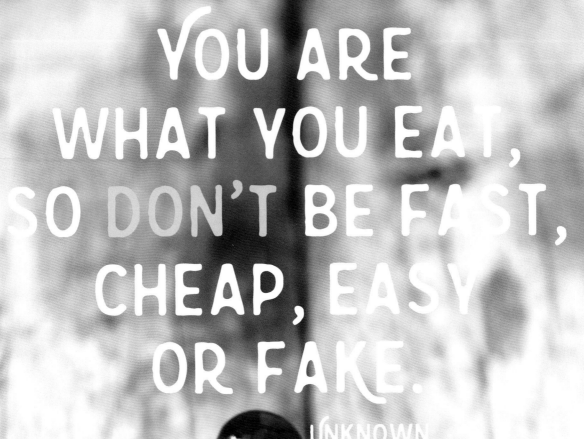

You are
what you eat,
so don't be fast,
cheap, easy
or fake.

UNKNOWN

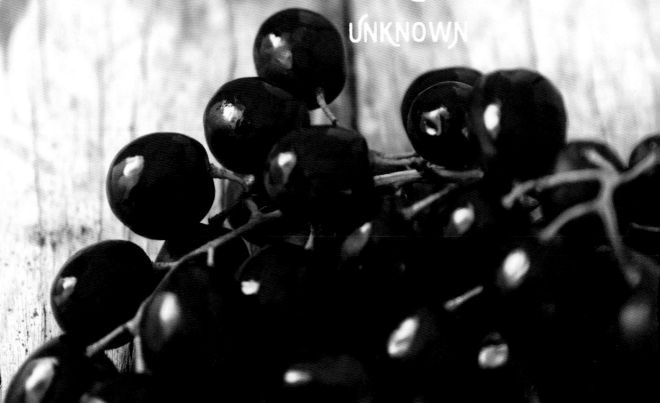

GOOD MORNING LOVELY PEOPLE,
LET'S MAKE IT A GREAT DAY!

My morning routine has remained pretty locked in since I changed my eating habits many years ago. I drink plenty of water on waking, slip into my workout gear, make a green juice or blend, pour it into a flask or bottle and head to the gym. I then drink my juice in the sauna after the workout and BOOM, I'm ready for the day! This clearly varies, as doing exactly the same thing every day isn't my thing (I get bored extremely easily!) but the essence of my morning remains the same; Up, Water, Workout and Juice. I like to do this as it keeps me feeling light and sharp, setting me up beautifully for the day ahead. Equally though, I also like to mix it up – especially at weekends — when I'll have something other than a juice or blend. However, whatever I choose to break my overnight fast with, I make certain it's nutritionally sound and tastes 'off the chart' amazing. As breakfast is roughly a third of what you are going to consume in a day and therefore a lifetime, it's worth getting it right!

This is why, along with some of my favorite morning Super-Blends, for a 'break on the go', I've included some breakfasts you can actually get your teeth (and knife and fork) into.

Other dishes in this section include:

- KATIE'S SUPERFOOD PORRIDGE (page 49)
- JASON'S GORGEOUS GRANOLA (page 51)
- JASEY'S SUPERFOOD MUESLI (page 53)
- FREE-RANGE, SUPER-CHARGED SCRAMBLED EGGS ON RYE (page 59)
- HERBACEOUS OMELETTE WITH GRILLED CHERRY TOMATOES (page 61)
- THE EASY ENGLISH – BREAKFAST IN A BAKING TRAY! (page 63)

I have also included some wonderful alternatives to cow's milk to go with your homemade **superfood** muesli and porridge, including Almond Milk (page 55), Banana Milk (page 57) and even Mixed Seed Milk (page 57).

Remember to snap a pic of whichever breakfast you make and share it on social media to spread the Super *fast* Food message and help to make a difference.

#superfastfood

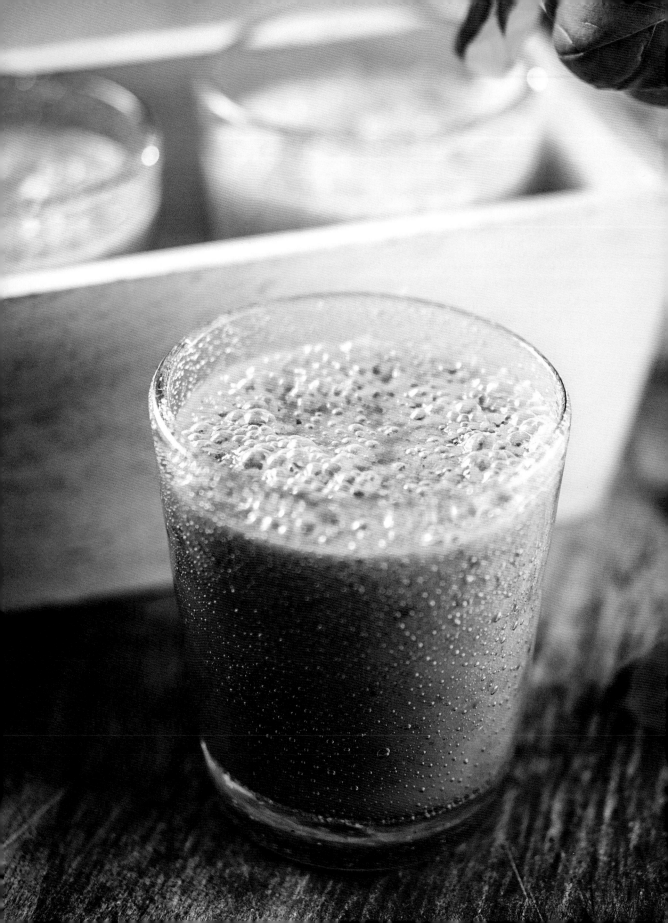

GLUTEN-FREE

VEGAN

VEGETARIAN

WAKE UP, SHAKE UP!

NO JUICER REQUIRED — JUST BLEND & GO!

Four or five days a week you'll see me break my overnight sleeping fast with a juice or smoothie of some kind, and when I'm in a rush, Wake Up, Shake Up! does the job beautifully. Despite this breakfast being in liquid form, don't get it confused with a drink. This is very much a 'complete breakfast' in a glass and one of the most nutritious you'll ever have. The naturally refreshing juice from cucumber acts as a diuretic, removing bloating caused by excess water retention. Cucumber is also wonderful for the hair, nails and skin. Avocado is perhaps the best superfood on earth and contains all seven human nutritional needs — protein, fats, carbohydrates, vitamins, minerals, water and enzymes. The pear adds good fibre to help get things 'moving' first thing, as well as some natural sweetness, whilst the basil lifts the whole 'dish' and just adds that little extra something.

INGREDIENTS:

Serves 2

Pears
2 medium

Basil
20g or 2 small handfuls

Cucumber
6cm or 2 small chunks

Avocado (ripe)
1 small

Filtered Water
500ml / 18 fl oz

Ice
a few cubes

PREPARE:

Cut the pear in quarters, remove the core and chop into small pieces. Remove the leaves from the basil and discard the stalks. Chop the cucumber into small pieces. Remove the flesh from the avocado.

BLEND:

Add all the ingredients to a blender or a *Retro Super Blend* and blend for 30 — 60 seconds.

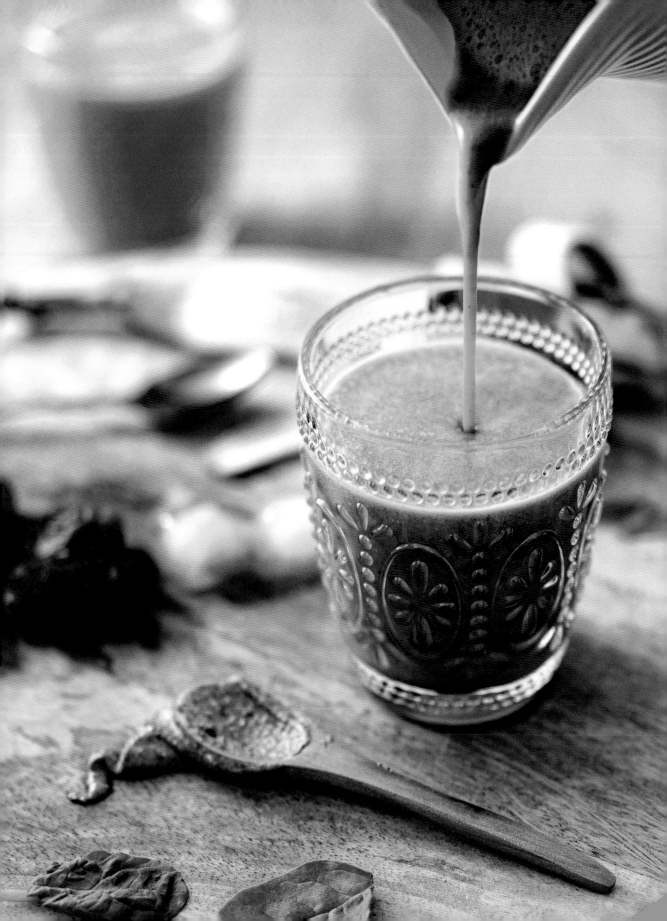

SPIRULINA SUPER BLEND

LIQUID SUPERFOOD BREAKFAST!

The title of this book is Super *fast* Food and this pure liquid 'breakfast on the go' fits that title beautifully. It's a superfood breakfast made in less than a couple of minutes. The banana provides a good source of fibre, is low in salt and high in potassium. Bananas are officially recognized by the FDA as being able to lower blood pressure and protect against heart attacks and strokes; just in case taste wasn't reason enough to get some into your body! Almond butter is rich in good fats and amino acids, the building blocks for protein. The dates add that wonderful sweetness to counteract the bitter flavors of the spinach and spirulina, as well as having good pedigree when it comes to breaking a fast. Medjool dates have been used to break the fast of Ramadan since ancient times. Spirulina is one of the richest natural sources of protein on earth and, like the dates, is abundant in iron. All round it's one hell of a Super *fast* Food breakfast and if you're into your 'protein shakes' then skip the powders and replace with this bad boy!

INGREDIENTS:

Serves 2

Dates (Medjool are so yummy)
4
Banana (Fair Trade)
1
Almond Nut Butter
2 generous teaspoons
Spinach
100g or 2 handfuls
Spirulina
2 level teaspoons
Filtered Water
500ml / 18 fl oz
Ice
a few cubes

PREPARE:

Remove any hard ends and the stones from the dates, chop into small pieces. Peel the banana.

BLITZ:

Place all the ingredients into the blender or *Retro Super Blend* and blast for 30 — 60 seconds.

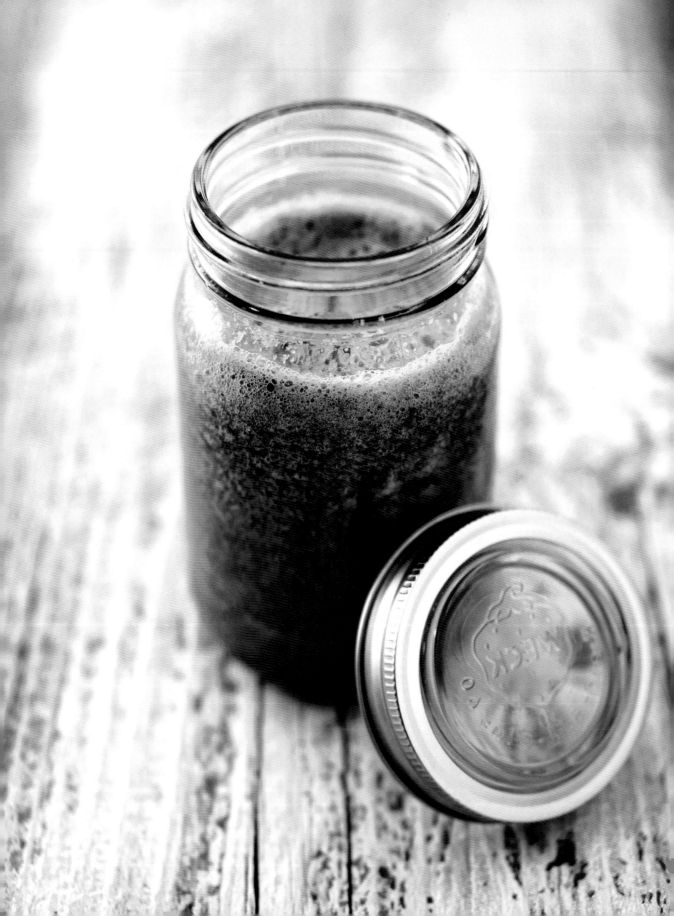

MINTY COCONUT SUPER BREAKFAST BLAST
BREAKFAST ON THE GO

GLUTEN-FREE

VEGAN

VEGETARIAN

If an 'apple a day keeps the doctor away' then by adding some fresh mint, a bit of banana, a handful of spinach and some coconut water, the chances are he'll never come knocking again! It not only wins many prizes on the health front, but it tastes ridiculously good too. Coconut water and banana are a natural match made in heaven, but add the mint and you take it to another level. Rich in fiber, vitamins, minerals, amino acids, and good natural carbs, this incredibly super fast to make superfood breakfast will provide you with enough energy to see you through till lunch (unless you're an elite athlete and start your day with a 20 mile run. If that's the case I'd suggest perhaps following up with the Free-Range, Super-Charged Scrambled Eggs on Rye page 59).

INGREDIENTS:

Serves 2

Apples
2
Fresh Mint
20g or 2 small handfuls
Banana (Fair Trade)
1
Spinach
100g or 2 handfuls
Coconut Water
400ml / 14 fl oz
Ice
a few cubes

PREPARE:

Remove the core from the apple and chop into small pieces. Remove the leaves from the mint and discard the stems. Peel the banana.

WHIZZ:

Place everything in a blender or *Retro Super Blend* and whizz for 30 — 60 seconds.

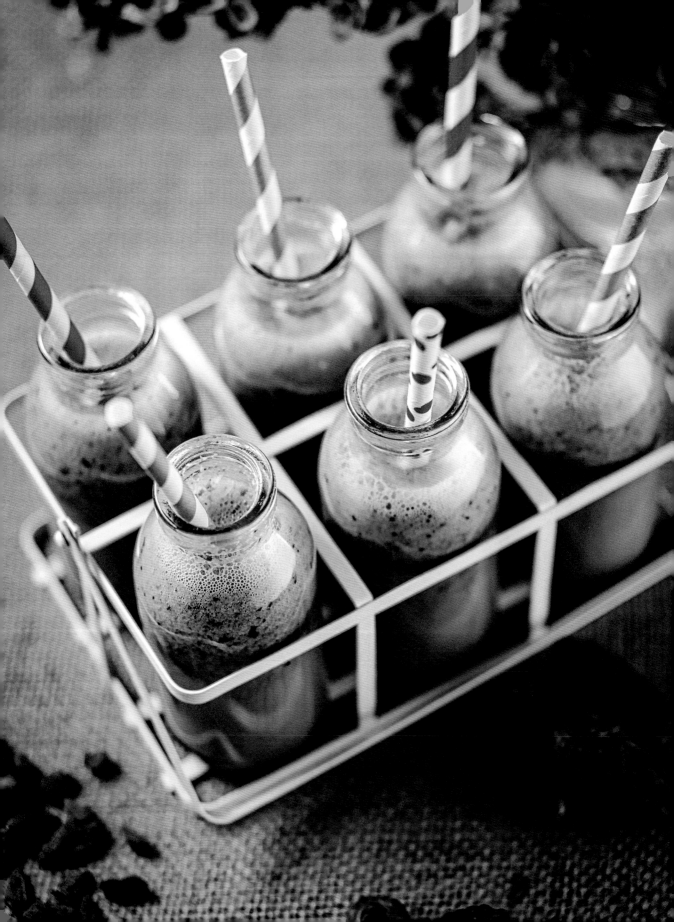

ANTIOXIDANT BERRY BLAST
GOOD MORNING JUICY PEOPLE

This is it; the super blend of all super blends. If this doesn't rock your taste buds, nothing will. As the name suggests it's perhaps the richest antioxidant super blend I have ever devised. Berries are widely regarded as the antioxidant 'kings' of the fruit world and none more so than the new berry on the block — goji! I say new, but you can now get goji berries pretty much anywhere (well not in B&Q but you get the idea). Goji berries are the most nutritionally dense fruit on earth and are rich in vitamin C, vitamin B2, vitamin A, iron, selenium and many other antioxidants. It is said they contain twice as many antioxidants as blueberries and blueberries were already considered top of the berry list in that genre. If you can't get hold of all of the berries in question, you can make with just one type or whatever you have. However, for full nutritional and taste value, stick to the recipe if you can. The almond milk tones down the sweetness beautifully and makes for one of the creamiest super blends you'll ever taste. If it's a nice fruit boost you want first thing, then this little baby is what you're looking for!

INGREDIENTS:

Serves 2

Almond or Seed Milk
500ml / 18 fl oz
(see pages 53 & 55)

Dates (Medjool are the best)
4

Goji Berries
20g or 2 small handfuls

Blackberries*
80g or 2 small handfuls

Blueberries*
40g or 2 small handfuls

Raspberries*
40g or 2 small handfuls

Ice*
a few cubes

DAY BEFORE PREP:

You will need almond or seed milk for this recipe, so please go to pages 55 & 57 as you will need to soak your almonds or seeds the day before to make the milk.

PREPARE!

Remove any hard ends and stones from the dates and chop.

BLAST:

Add all the ingredients to the blender and blast up for 30 – 60 seconds.

*You can use fresh or frozen berries. If you use frozen, then skip the ice, or your smoothie will end up like a Slush Puppy!

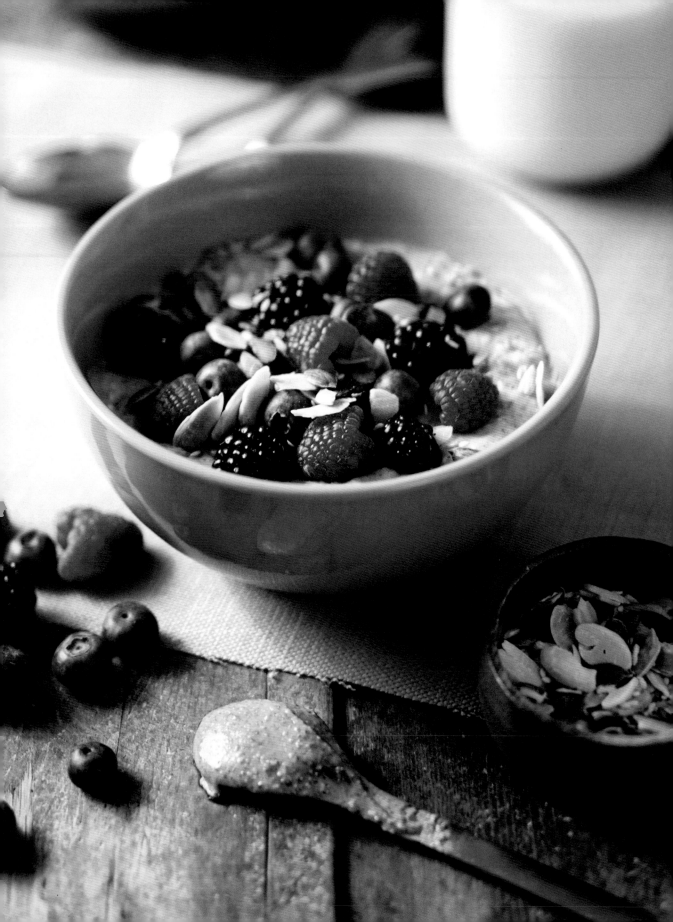

KATIE'S SUPERFOOD PORRIDGE
ALMOND & GINGER INFUSED PORRIDGE
WITH TOASTED NUTS, SEEDS & BERRIES

GLUTEN-FREE

VEGAN

VEGETARIAN

CONTAINS NUTS

There's porridge and then there's this beauty! I remember porridge growing up and it was more 'super bland' than superfood. Oats on their own, even with just hot water, could indeed be classed as a superfood but it tastes a little of cardboard (not that I've eaten cardboard, so I'm just guessing!) However, it doesn't take a great deal to take this classic brekkie to another level on the taste and nutrition front and my lovely Katie, who has more than helped with this book, has made this her own. The combination of fresh almond milk, almond butter and oats creates a creaminess to die for, whilst the fresh berries add the sweetness you want on top of porridge. The ginger gives a nice unexpected kick, while the seeds provide good fats in abundance. If you haven't tasted porridge for a while because it's usually too 'blah'. then may I introduce to you Katie's Superfood Porridge, you'll be very pleased you made its acquaintance.

INGREDIENTS:

Serves 2

Ginger
approx. 40g or 4 x 4cm

Flaked Almonds
25g or 1 small handful

Mixed Seeds
25g or 1 small handful

Rolled Oats*
100g or 7 tablespoons

Almond Milk
500ml / 18 fl oz (see page 55)

Himalayan Rock Salt
1 pinch

Almond Butter
1 tablespoon

Fresh Berries
(any sort, you decide)
100g or 1 large handful

DAY BEFORE PREP:

For best results and optimum nutrition, soak the almonds over night so they are ready to use tomorrow to make the almond milk (page 55).

PREPARE:

Preheat the oven to 180 °C (350 °F / gas mark 4).

Peel the ginger and grate using a small hand grater.

COOK:

Place the flaked almonds and seeds onto a baking tray and pop in the oven for 5 minutes. Meanwhile, put the oats, almond milk, ginger and salt in a pan, gently bring to the boil, then reduce the heat and cook for 2 – 3 minutes, stirring constantly. Remove from the heat, add the almond butter and stir well.

SERVE:

Spoon the porridge into a bowl, add the fresh berries and finish with the toasted almonds and seeds.

*Oats are technically gluten-free but unfortunately some commercial oats have been cross contaminated with wheat, barley or rye, during the harvesting, storage, milling or processing, so be a little careful here if you are particularly sensitive.

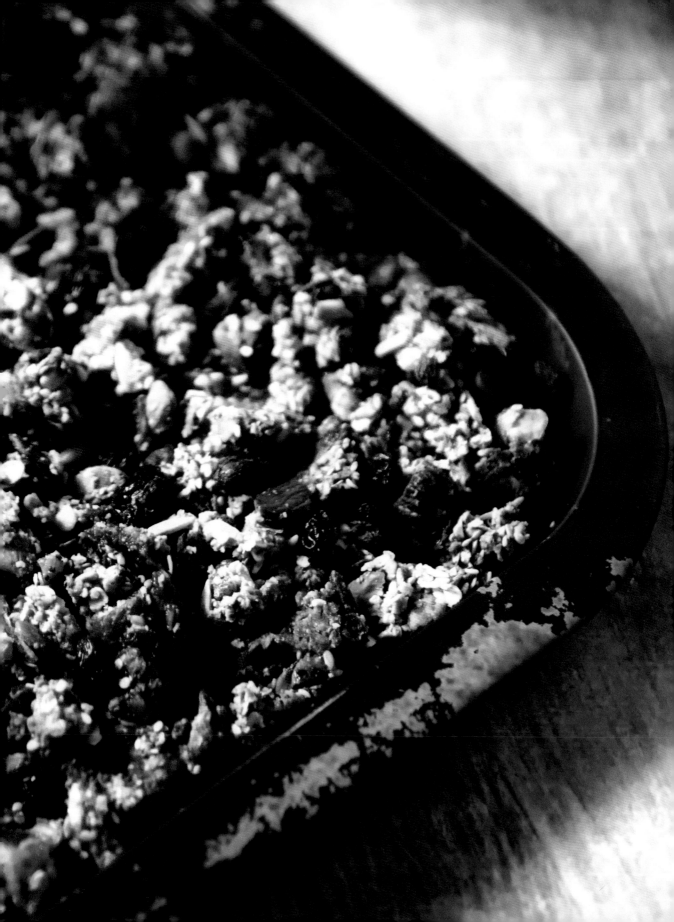

JASEY'S SUPERFOOD GRANOLA

The book says 'fast food' in the title and you may feel you need to get in the trades description folks here. However, before you pick up the phone, this recipe makes an entire batch. In other words once you've made it, it will last for weeks – especially if you are juicing or super blending for other days. So although it takes a little longer than the other breakfasts to make initially, once done, it then becomes super fast the rest of the time. Plus, once you taste this absolutely 'out the park' granola, you won't actually care how long it took you to make it — yes even if I do say so myself, it's that good!

GLUTEN-FREE

VEGAN

VEGETARIAN

CONTAINS NUTS

INGREDIENTS:

Makes approx. 600g / 21oz

Dates (Medjool are 'king' of dates)
8

Filtered Water
100ml / 3.5 fl oz

Apricots (un-sulphured if possible)
80g or 1 large handful

Almonds
100g or 2 handfuls

Goji Berries
70g or 1 large handful

Mixed Seeds
100g / 3.5oz

Poppy Seeds
20g or 1 small handful

Oats*
100g or 7 tablespoons

Nutmeg
½ teaspoon

Coconut Oil
15ml or 1 tablespoon

Honey**
30ml or 2 tablespoons

Raisins
70g or 1 large handful

PREP THE DAY BEFORE:

Remove any hard ends and stones from the dates and chop each one into quarters. Place in a container and cover with the water, leaving overnight or for a minimum of 2 hours. If you are going to serve the granola with gorgeous almond, banana or seed milk, then make sure you soak the almonds or seeds today as well (see pages 55 & 57).

PREPARE:

Preheat the oven to 150 °C (300 °F / gas mark 2).

Place the dates and the water in a mixing bowl. Coarsely chop the apricots and almonds and add to the mixing bowl, along with the goji berries, mixed seeds, poppy seeds, oats and nutmeg. Gently combine.

COOK:

Put the coconut oil and honey on a baking tray and place in the oven for 1 minute. Pour the granola mixture onto the baking tray, distribute evenly and bake for 40 minutes, stirring part way through. Remove from the oven, add the raisins and allow to cool. Store in an airtight container.

The granola should easily last for a couple of weeks, but whether it actually will or not is another matter, as it's never around for long in our house!

SERVE:

Best served with banana, seed or almond milk (see pages 55 & 57) or even with some live yogurt and a drizzle of honey.

*Oats are technically gluten-free but unfortunately some commercial oats have been cross contaminated with wheat, barley or rye, during the harvesting, storage, milling or processing, so be a little careful here if you are particularly sensitive.

**If vegan, please use an alternative sweetener

FACTOID

Both muesli and granola contain very similar ingredients. The key difference is that granola is often sweetened and then baked, whereas muesli is served raw/uncooked.

JASEY'S SUPERFOOD MUESLI

NUTTY, SEEDED, CINNAMON & CRANBERRY MUESLI

GLUTEN-FREE

VEGAN

VEGETARIAN

CONTAINS NUTS

My beautiful mother was obsessed with muesli for breakfast when I was growing up, but the challenge was the added refined sugar. This is why I now make my own. Not only am I in full control of everything that goes in it, but it's also much cheaper. This recipe makes the equivalent of a box of cereal, so once you've made it, store in a lovely large jar and it's then ready for whenever you are! Feel free to add fresh berries when in season, like black, blue or straw and a little freshly chopped banana never goes amiss when you want to mix it up. Loaded with nutrients, packed with flavour and a great way to start the day!

INGREDIENTS:

Makes approx. 575g / 20oz

Pecan Nuts
50g or 1 handful

Almonds
50g or 1 handful

Blanched Hazelnuts
50g or 1 handful

Rolled Oats*
150g or 10 tablespoons

Dried Cranberries
75g or 1 large handful

Raisins
50g or 1 handful

Mixed Seeds
100g / 4oz

Ground Almonds
50g / 2oz

Ground Cinnamon
1 teaspoon

DAY BEFORE PREP:

If you are going to serve with beautiful almond, banana or seed milk, then don't forget to soak the almonds/seeds today (see pages 55 & 57).

PREPARE:

Finely chop the pecan, almond and hazelnuts, leaving a few larger pieces. Place the nuts and all the other ingredients into a mixing bowl, stir, then store in an airtight container.

SERVE:

Best served with any of the milks found on pages 55 & 57.

*Oats are technically gluten-free but unfortunately some commercial oats have been cross contaminated with wheat, barley or rye, during the harvesting, storage, milling or processing, so be a little careful here if you are particularly sensitive.

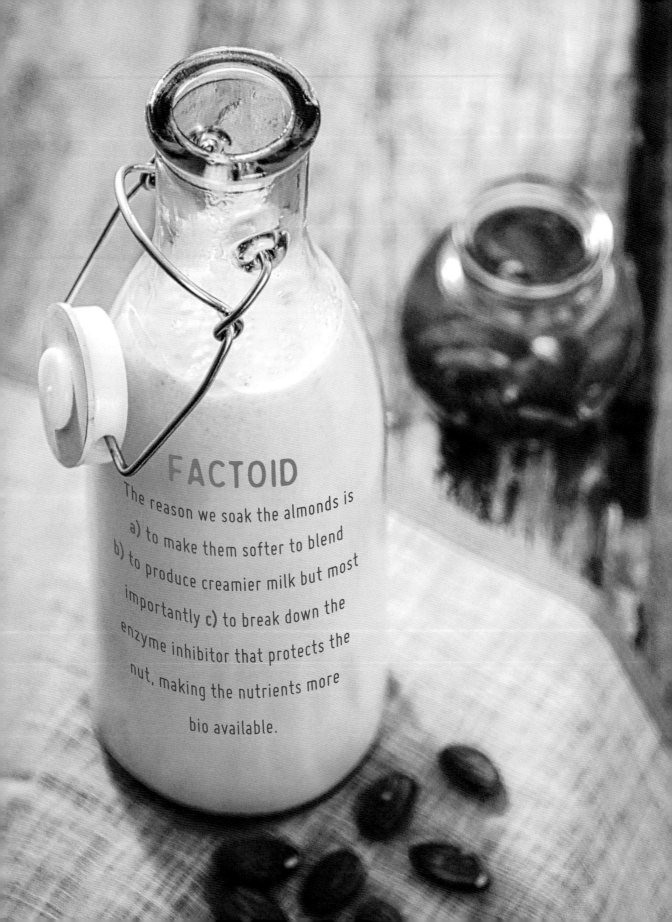

FACTOID

The reason we soak the almonds is a) to make them softer to blend b) to produce creamier milk but most importantly c) to break down the enzyme inhibitor that protects the nut, making the nutrients more bio available.

SUPER MILKS

Growing up I suffered with severe psoriasis, eczema and asthma. My asthma was so bad that I used my asthma pump over fourteen times daily and my skin conditions were so extreme that I couldn't even wear jeans without my skin cracking (hope I haven't put you off your breakfast!?) Medical drugs and creams had no effect and it wasn't until I removed dairy from my world that things started to improve. I am not a doctor so please don't take this as a 'go dairy free and you'll be cured' message, because it isn't. However, I have seen hundreds of people for whom a departure from dairy has resulted in good improvements in these conditions. Here are 3 alternatives to dairy; my personal number 1 go to is almond milk. Unlike dairy and some other nuts milks, it is alkalising rather than acidic. Almond milk also contains vitamin D, calcium, vitamin E and is low carb meaning it has little impact on blood sugar levels. As well as being better for you (in my opinion) than cow's milk, it tastes better!

ALMOND MILK

DAY BEFORE PREP
+
ROUGHLY 3-4 MINS

INGREDIENTS:

Makes 1 litre

Almonds
100g or 2 handfuls
Tap Water
200ml / 7 fl oz
Filtered Water
800ml / 28 fl oz
Himalayan Rock Salt
1 pinch

PREP THE DAY BEFORE:

Soak the almonds in the tap water overnight or for a minimum of 6 hours.

OPTION 1- MAKE WITH A BLENDER

Discard the almond water and rinse the almonds. Place the almonds, filtered water and salt into a blender or *Retro Super Blend* and blend for 1 — 2 minutes (depending on the power of your blender). Then pour the blended almonds through either a nut bag* or a sieve and voilà, you have almond milk!

OPTION 2- MAKE WITH A SLOW JUICER**

The newest addition to my kitchen is one of the beautiful 'Retro' upright slow juicers. I heard on the grapevine that you could use a slow juicer to make almond milk, so I set the Retro to task and not only does it work, but it's also stupidly simple and fuss free. All you do is add a quarter of the soaked nuts, turn the juicer on, gradually pour about 200ml / 7 fl oz of the filtered water through, then add another quarter of nuts and a further 200ml / 7 fl oz of water and so on until all the nuts and water have been used. Then bingo, creamy almond milk flows from one shoot and dried almond 'flour' pops out of the other. Lastly, sprinkle the rock salt into the milk and give it a quick stir and enjoy!

GOOD TO KNOW:

- The almond milk will keep in the fridge for up to 3 days.
- Over time the milk will separate slightly due to the natural fats, so simply give it a stir before you use it.
- As an alternative you can use other nuts such as brazil nuts or hazelnuts.

* Nut bags are widely available online
** Please note you cannot make nut milk with a 'fast' or centrifugal juicer. You have been warned!

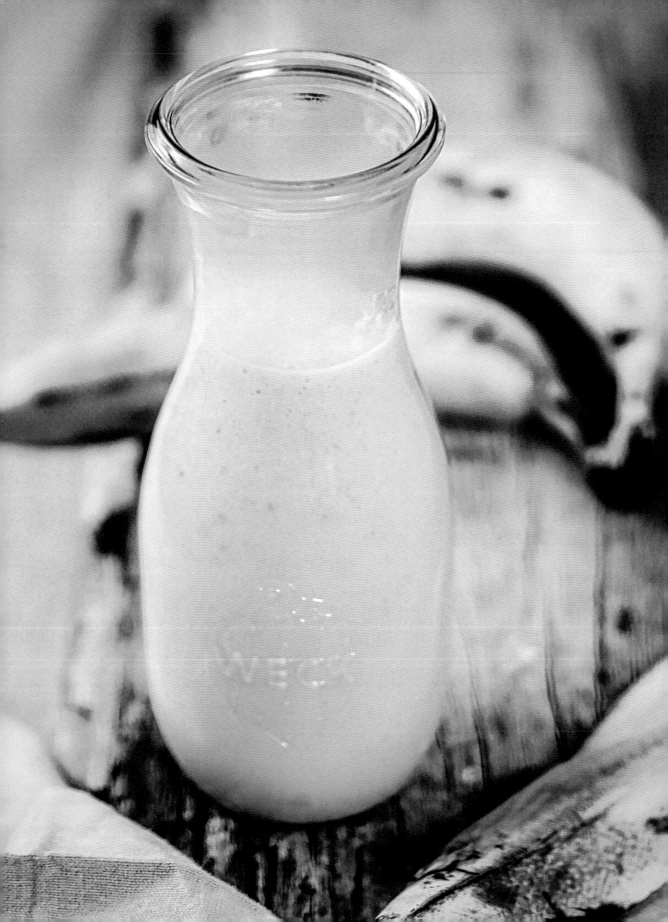

BANANA MILK (SHOWN)

GLUTEN-FREE

VEGAN

VEGETARIAN

CONTAINS NUTS

INGREDIENTS:

Makes 300 ml / 10.5 fl oz

Almond Milk
200ml / 7 fl oz (see page 53)

Banana (Fair Trade)
1

MAKE:

Blend the almond milk and banana for 30 — 60 seconds and then drink straight away (if you prefer a thicker 'milk shake' drink, leave for 30 — 60 minutes in the fridge) — In the words of Porky Pig... 'Tha-Tha-Tha-Tha-That's all folks'!

MIXED SEED MILK

GLUTEN-FREE

VEGAN

VEGETARIAN

CONTAINS NUTS

INGREDIENTS:

Makes 1 litre

Mixed Seeds
100g / 4oz

Tap Water
200ml / 7 fl oz

Filtered Water
800ml / 28 fl oz

Himalayan Rock Salt
1 pinch

Honey**
1 tablespoon

DAY BEFORE PREP:

Soak the seeds in the tap water overnight or for a minimum of 6 hours.

MAKE:

Pour away the water and rinse the seeds. Place the seeds, filtered water, salt and honey into a blender or *Retro Super Blend* and blend for 1 — 2 minutes (depending on the power of your blender). Pour the blended seed mixture through either a nut bag* or a sieve and discard the pulp. Boom, delicious seed milk in minutes!

JUST SO YOU KNOW:

- The seed milk will keep in the fridge for up to 3 days.

- The milk will separate quite quickly, but do not worry; this is simply due to the oils from the seeds combining with the water. Before you use it, simply give it a little stir.

* Nut bags are widely available online

** If vegan please use an alternative sweetener.

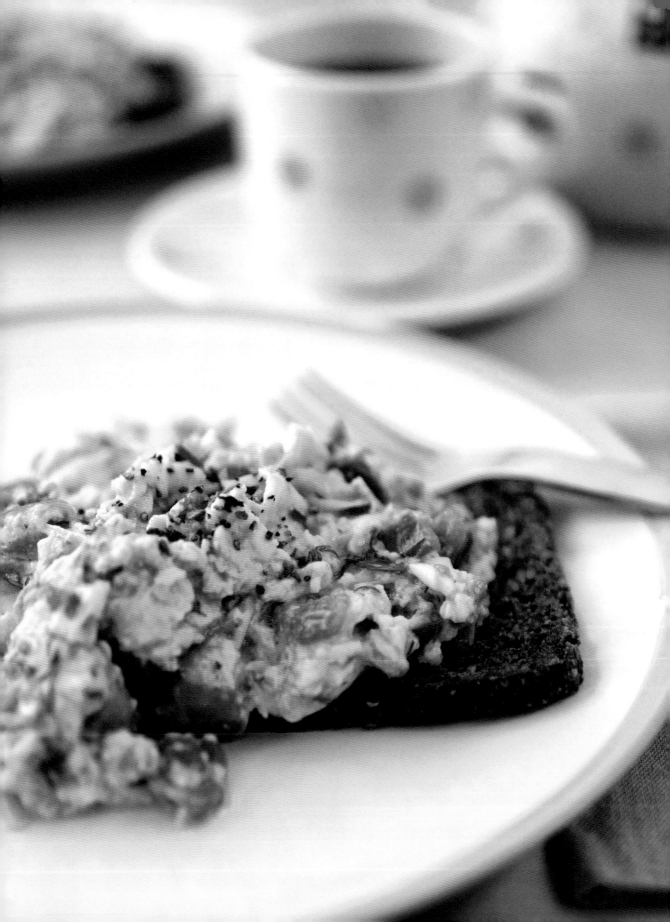

VEGETARIAN

FREE-RANGE, SUPER-CHARGED SCRAMBLED EGGS ON RYE

I LOVE eggs, there I said it; it's now out in the open! Eggs are perhaps the most versatile of all superfoods. They are packed with high quality protein, a rich source of selenium, vitamins A, D, E, B6, B12 and minerals such as zinc, iron and copper, so worthy of the superfood title. Eggs are also the cheapest of all superfoods and you won't have to go to an obscure shop in the back streets of Notting Hill to get hold of them! These Super-Charged Scrambled Eggs are my staple on a Sunday morning and I hope they find a place in your world too. Bursting with flavour, loaded with macro and micronutrients and incredibly filling, this breakfast hits just about every button.

INGREDIENTS:

Serves 2

Eggs (free-range & organic)
6 large

Spring Onions
2 Stalks

Tomatoes
200g or 3 medium

Fresh Dill
10g or 1 small handful

Olive Oil
½ tablespoon

Rye Bread*
2 large or 4 small slices

Ground Black Pepper
1 generous pinch

Himalayan Rock Salt
1 pinch

Butter
A couple of knobs or you could use coconut oil

PREPARE:

Crack the eggs into a bowl and whisk.

Remove the outer layer and ends from the spring onions and thinly slice diagonally (they look better this way!). Chop the tomatoes into small cubes. Remove any hard stalks from the dill and finely chop.

COOK:

Put the oil into a frying pan and warm over a medium to high heat. Add the spring onion and tomatoes and cook for 3 minutes, stirring occasionally. Whilst the mixture is cooking, toast the rye bread. Reduce to a medium heat, add the eggs, dill and seasoning and allow to cook for 2 – 3 minutes, stirring constantly until the eggs are *almost* cooked. Remove from the heat and continue to stir, as the eggs will continue to cook. Most of the moisture should have disappeared, but the mixture should still be lovely and moist.

SERVE:

Butter the toasted rye bread and cover with the gorgeous scrambled egg.

DID YOU KNOW...

There is a misconception that you need butter and milk to make creamy scrambled eggs. However it's more than possible to create creamy eggs; the secret is to cook them over a low heat for longer as opposed to quickly cooking them over a high heat.

*Rye bread is optional and this dish is equally as great just on its own.

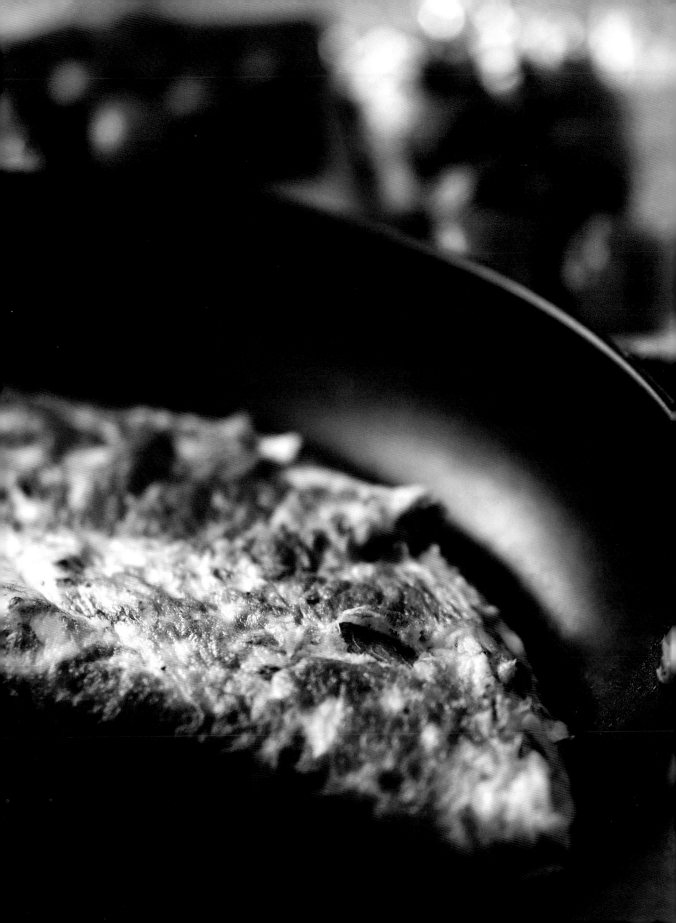

HERBACEOUS OMELETTE
WITH GRILLED CHERRY TOMATOES

GLUTEN-FREE

VEGETARIAN

Not all omelettes are built the same and some are better than others — this is one of them! As the name suggests, the herbs are the stars of the show here and raise the already superfood status of eggs to another level. Rich in vitamins A, E, B6 and B12, an excellent source of protein, natural fats and it's also worth knowing that eggs contain more vitamin D than they did 10 years ago, which helps to protect bones, preventing osteoporosis and rickets. Served on its own or with a couple of cheeky grilled tomatoes and veggie sausages (see Veggie Bangers 'n' Mash page 185) it will be one of the breakfasts I guarantee you'll return to time and time again.

INGREDIENTS:

Serves 2

Fresh Mint
10g or 1 small handful

Fresh Basil
10g or 1 small handful

Fresh Thyme
10g or 1 small handful

Fresh Coriander
10g or 1 small handful

Eggs (free-range and organic)
6 large

Ground Black Pepper
1 generous pinch

Almond Milk or Crème Fraîche
30 ml or 2 tablespoons

Cherry Tomatoes (on the vine)
120g or 10

Olive oil
1 tablespoon

PREPARE:

Preheat the grill. Place a piece of tin foil on a small baking tray. Remove the leaves from the mint and basil and discard the stalks. Finely chop the mint, basil, thyme and coriander. Break the eggs into a mixing bowl, add the pepper and almond milk or crème fraîche and whisk for about 30 seconds. Then add the herbs and mix for a few more seconds.

COOK:

Place the cherry tomatoes (still on the vine if possible) on the baking tray and pop under the grill for 4 – 5 minutes until cooked. Meanwhile drizzle half of the olive oil into the frying pan and place over a medium to high heat, then add half the egg mixture and tilt the pan, so the bottom of the pan is covered. Allow to cook for 2 – 3 minutes, until the omelette just starts to form, then fold in half and cook for a further 30 seconds. Pop on a plate with half of the tomatoes and serve to your loved one, whilst you repeat the above and cook the second omelette.

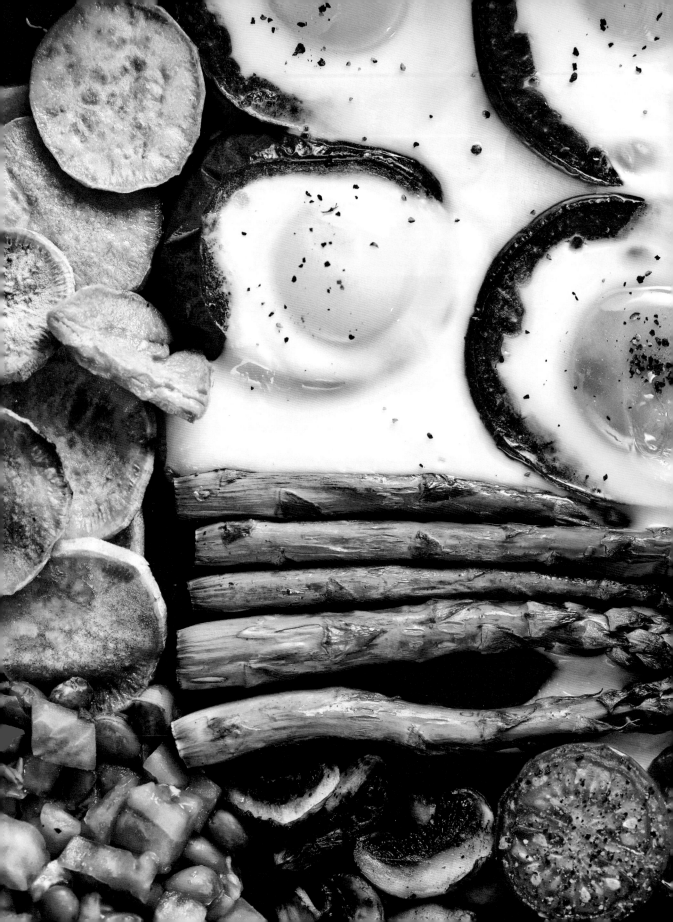

GLUTEN-FREE

VEGETARIAN

THE EASY ENGLISH – BREAKFAST IN A BAKING TRAY!

The main problem with a traditional English breakfast is the number of pans you use and consequently the number that then need washing up. The other issue is timing, which is why I have created a breakfast that only uses one baking tray, so it's quick to make and wash up! This is a tasty, healthy and most importantly, an easy breakfast to rustle up. You'll see I have missed out the homemade vegetarian sausages simply due to the amount of time this would add on. However if you do have any sausages (bought or premade) in the freezer, then add them instead of the sweet potato. If you simply must have some meat, then feel free to substitute the sweet potato with a 'real' sausage, but I assure you, this version will leave you feeling very satisfied.

INGREDIENTS:

Serves 2

Beef Tomato
1 large
Tomatoes
150g or 2 medium
Mushrooms
100g or 4 medium
Asparagus
140g or 8 spears
Sweet Potato
1 medium
Borlotti Beans
200g or ½ can
Olive Oil
2 tablespoons
Himalayan Rock Salt
2 pinches
Ground Black Pepper
2 generous pinches
Eggs (free-range & organic)
4 medium
Rye Bread (optional)
2 slices
Coconut Oil or Butter
a knob

PREPARE:

Preheat the oven to 200 °C (400 °F / gas mark 6). Slice the ends from the Beef tomato and cut into 4 nice slices (about 1 cm thick). Using a small knife remove the flesh from inside the tomato to create a ring. Chop this flesh into very small pieces and place in a bowl. Cut the other tomatoes in half. Wash and slice the mushrooms. Remove any hard ends from the asparagus. Remove the ends from the sweet potato, peel and thinly slice. Drain the water from the beans, rinse and then add to the bowl containing the tomato and mix.

COOK:

Drizzle ½ the olive oil over a large non-stick baking tray and place the mushroom, asparagus, sweet potato, beef tomato ring and the other halved tomatoes onto the baking tray. Drizzle the remaining olive oil over the mushrooms, asparagus and sweet potato and sprinkle the salt and pepper over the halved tomatoes.

Place in the oven and cook for 10 minutes. Then remove the baking tray from the oven, turn over the mushrooms, asparagus and potato and crack an egg into each of the tomato rings (don't worry if it spills over a little). Carefully replace the tray into the oven and cook for a further 7 minutes. Meanwhile if you want to add rye bread, pop it in the toaster. Remove the baking tray from the oven, add the bean and tomato mix and cook for a final 3 minutes.

SERVE:

Remove the tray from the oven, 'butter' the rye bread with the coconut oil or organic butter, arrange all the ingredients on your plate or eat straight out of the pan!

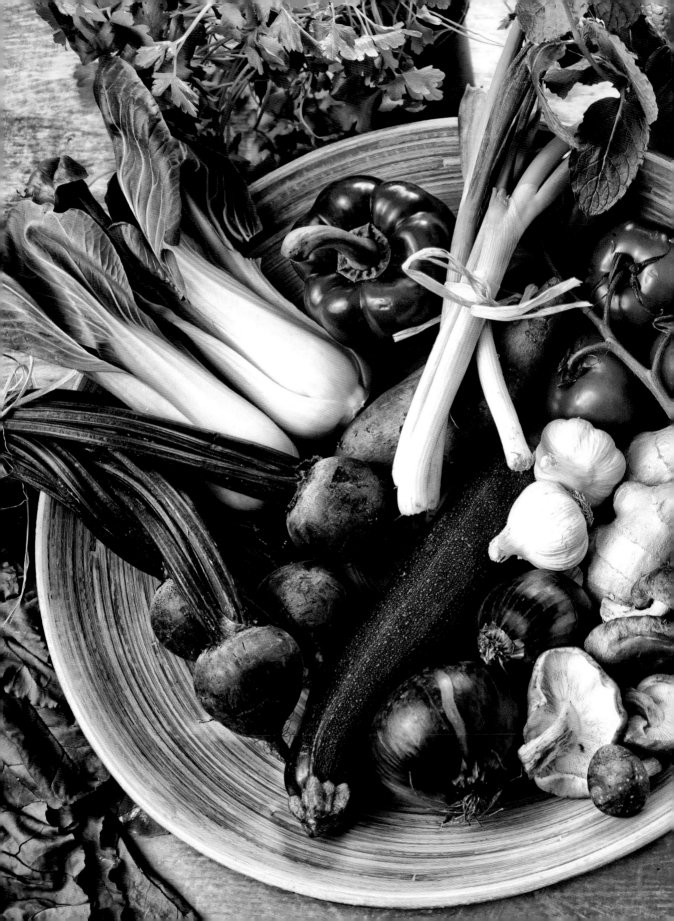

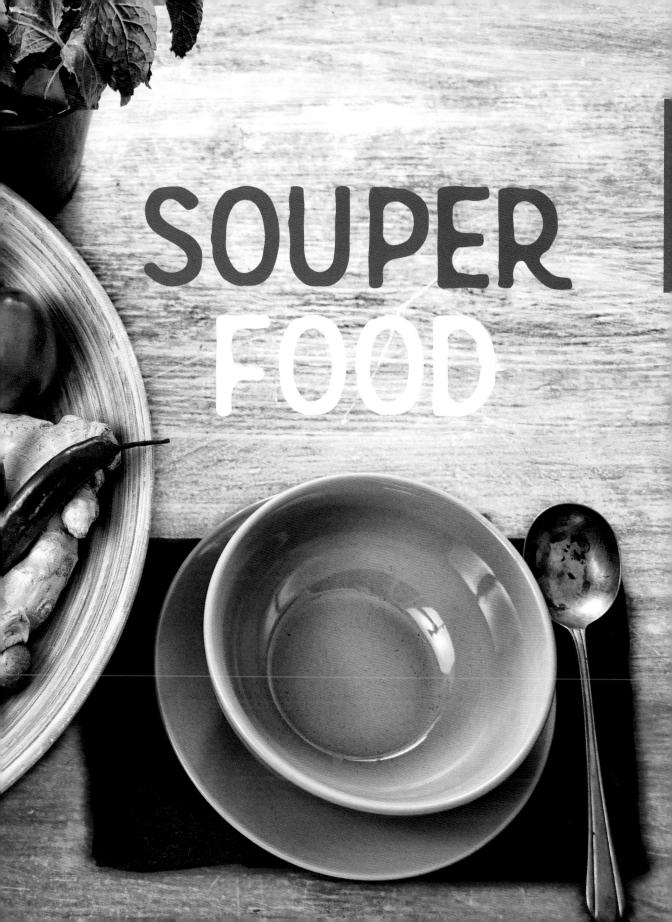

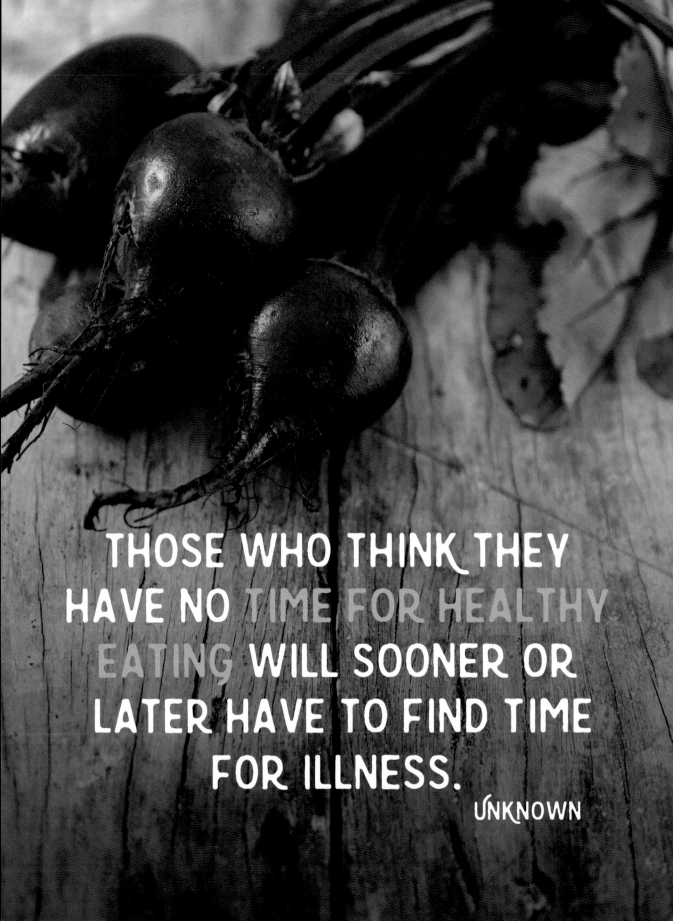

THOSE WHO THINK THEY HAVE NO TIME FOR HEALTHY EATING WILL SOONER OR LATER HAVE TO FIND TIME FOR ILLNESS.

UNKNOWN

SOUPER TASTY
SOUPER NUTRITIOUS
SOUPER FOOD

In my opinion, soups really don't get the taste or nutritional press they deserve and are often either completely overlooked or only get a showing when we're feeling unwell. This is partly due to canned soups being bland but also partly due to us thinking that a soup doesn't really constitute a meal. However, if this is you, I will tell you now, that once you've made the soups in this section it will completely transform your current soup perception. You'll realize from the moment that you take that first mouthful, a hearty soup can indeed be **off the scale** delicious and so filling that it more than meets the criteria of 'main course' status.

I have been an advocate of the humble soup for years and many people who do my 'juice challenges' often swap a juice for one of these beauties in the evening, especially if doing the challenge in the cold of winter. We even serve soups in the evenings at our 'juice' retreats during the winter months (much to everyone's approval!) and soups clearly play a huge part in my **Soup 'n' Juice Me! Plan**.

In this section you'll find four of the best;

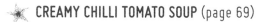 **CREAMY CHILLI TOMATO SOUP** (page 69)

COURGETTE, FENNEL & MINTY FRESH SOUP (page 71)

KATIE'S ORIENTAL SOUP..... WITH A KICK (page 73)

SWEET POTATO, BEETROOT & GINGER SOUP (page 75)

Each and every one as delicious and nutritionally thought through as the next, and each and every one worthy of their place within the pages of this **Super *fast* Food** book. Still not convinced? Then I would encourage you to make just one of these, try it and I pretty much guarantee you'll be converted for life. Also, by adding these to your diet you'll be doing yourself a massive favor on the health front as they're good to have before you get ill so you don't get ill!

Remember to snap a pic of whichever souper soup you decide to make and share it on social media to spread the **Super *fast* Food** message and help to make a difference.

#superfastfood

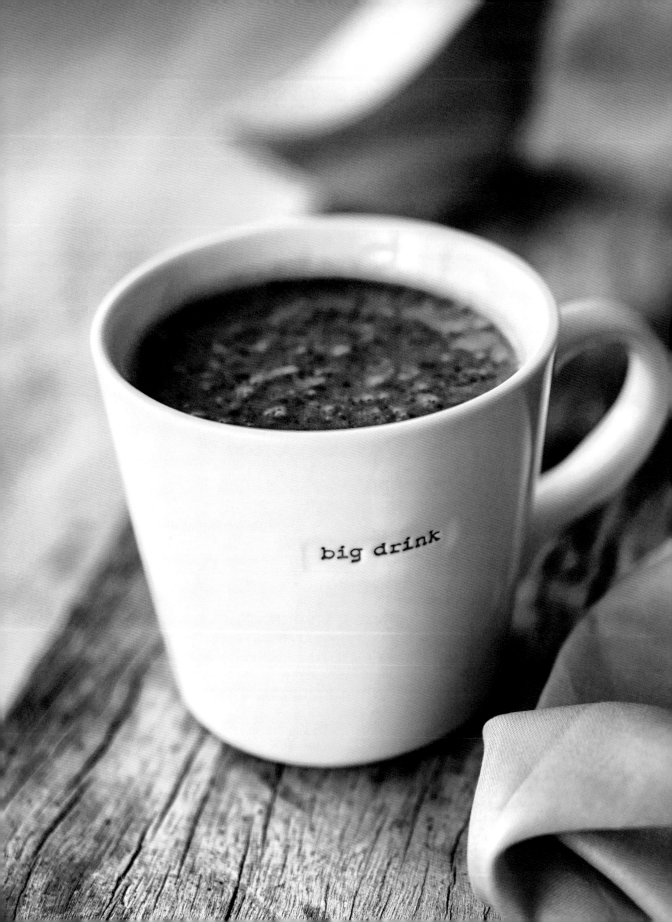

CREAMY CHILLI & TOMATO SOUP

If your idea of soup is something that you get in a can and consists of pretty much just tomato, then you are in for one hell of a treat with this bad boy. Not only does it live up nutritionally to the superfood mantel but it's honestly one of the nicest soups I've ever had. If you like a soup with a little kick, yet creamy to taste — you've found the one. This little soup is rich in protein; vitamins, minerals and the garlic and chilli add the 'Health Dr' element. Garlic is a natural antibiotic, natural anti-inflammatory and anti-fungal, whilst chilli peppers are a super rich source of vitamin C, with just 100g providing about 240% of our RDA. Vitamin C is required for collagen synthesis inside the human body. Collagen is one of the main structural proteins required for maintaining the integrity of blood vessels, skin, organs and bones. There are soups and then there's this taste bud dancing, nutrition busting Creamy Chilli & Tomato Soup.

GLUTEN-FREE

VEGAN

VEGETARIAN

INGREDIENTS:

Serves 2

Red Onion
½ medium
Red Pepper
½ medium
Red Chilli
2 medium
Garlic
2 cloves
Tomatoes
4 medium
Chilli Beans*
240g or 1 can
Coconut Oil or Olive Oil
1 tablespoon
Himalayan Rock Salt
1 pinch
Ground Black Pepper
1 good pinch
Boiling Water
200ml / 7 fl oz
Coconut Milk
200ml / 7 fl oz

PREPARE:

Remove the ends from the onion, peel and finely chop. Cut the red pepper in half, remove the seeds and chop into small pieces. Remove the ends from the chillis, chop in half lengthways, remove the seeds and chop into small pieces. Peel the garlic and thinly slice. Chop the tomato into small (ish) cubes. Drain and rinse the chilli beans.

COOK:

Put the coconut or olive oil in a large saucepan and warm over a moderate heat. Add the onion and red pepper and allow to soften for 5 minutes, stirring occasionally. Next add the chillis, garlic, tomatoes, chilli beans, salt and pepper. Reduce the heat and simmer for a further 5 minutes, then add the boiling water and coconut milk, allow to simmer for 2 minutes then remove from the heat.

BLEND:

Blend the soup for 1 — 2 minutes, using a stick blender or a regular blender. However **be extra careful** if opting for the latter as the build up of steam creates pressure that can force the lid off. Place a tea towel over the lid and hold down firmly whilst blending to avoid this.

SERVE:

Pour into a nice large mug or bowl and enjoy.

* If you prefer to use dry beans, then these will need soaking and cooking first, but it's perfectly ok to use pre-cooked beans from a can, just try and buy organic if possible.

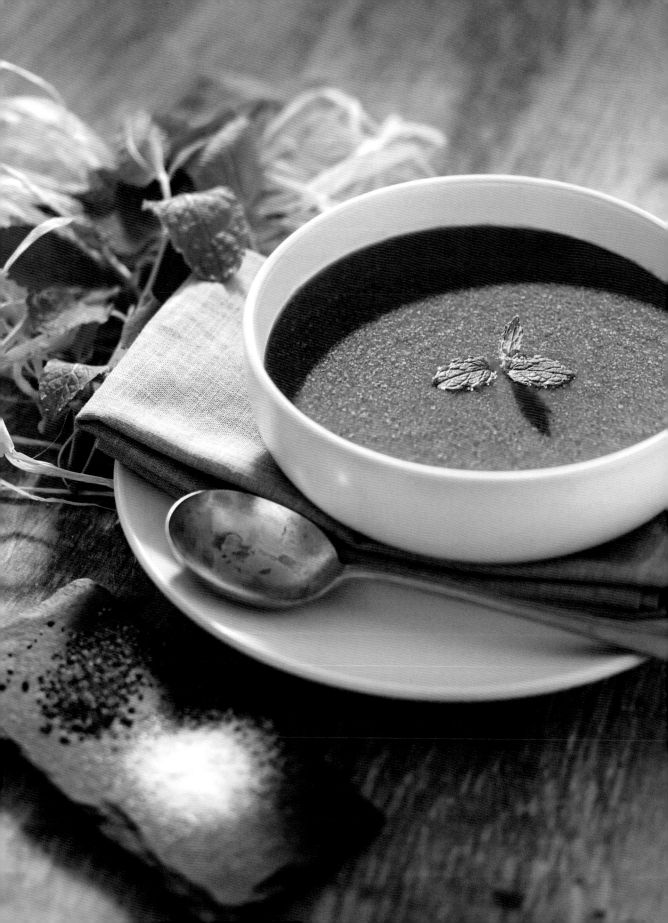

COURGETTE, FENNEL AND MINTY FRESH SOUP

GLUTEN-FREE

VEGAN

VEGETARIAN

Whenever I'm making a juice or soup I always like to add what I describe as a 'kicker' — something to lift it away from the 'vanilla' and into the world of interesting. The 'kickers' here are the fennel and mint. They lift beautifully what would otherwise be a fairly standard soup. Easy to make, packed with superfood nutrition such as the extremely vital vitamin C, antioxidants and an array of minerals. This little beaut once again hits the two buttons which are the theme of all recipes in this book — BIG on taste and BIG on nutrition!

INGREDIENTS:

Serves 2

Courgette/Zucchini
1 medium
Fennel
½ medium bulb
Celery
2 stalks
Fresh Mint
20g or 1 handful
Coconut Oil or Olive Oil
1 tablespoon
Himalayan Rock Salt
1 pinch
Ground Black Pepper
1 good pinch
Boiling Water
600 ml / 21 fl oz

PREPARE:

Remove the ends from the courgette/zucchini and fennel and then peel the courgette. Chop the courgette, fennel and celery into small (ish) slices. Remove the leaves from the mint and discard the stalks.

COOK:

Gently heat the coconut or olive oil in a pan over a medium heat and add the courgette, fennel and celery. Cook for 5 minutes, stirring occasionally until the vegetables start to soften, then add the salt, pepper and water, reduce the heat and continue to cook for a further 5 minutes.

BLEND:

Remove from the pan from the heat, add the fresh mint and blend for 1 — 2 minutes using either a stick blender or a regular blender. However **be very careful** if using a blender as the heat creates a build up of pressure that can blow the lid off!

Ensure you cover the lid with a tea towel and hold down firmly whilst blending to avoid this.

SERVE:

Pour the soup into a bowl and enjoy!

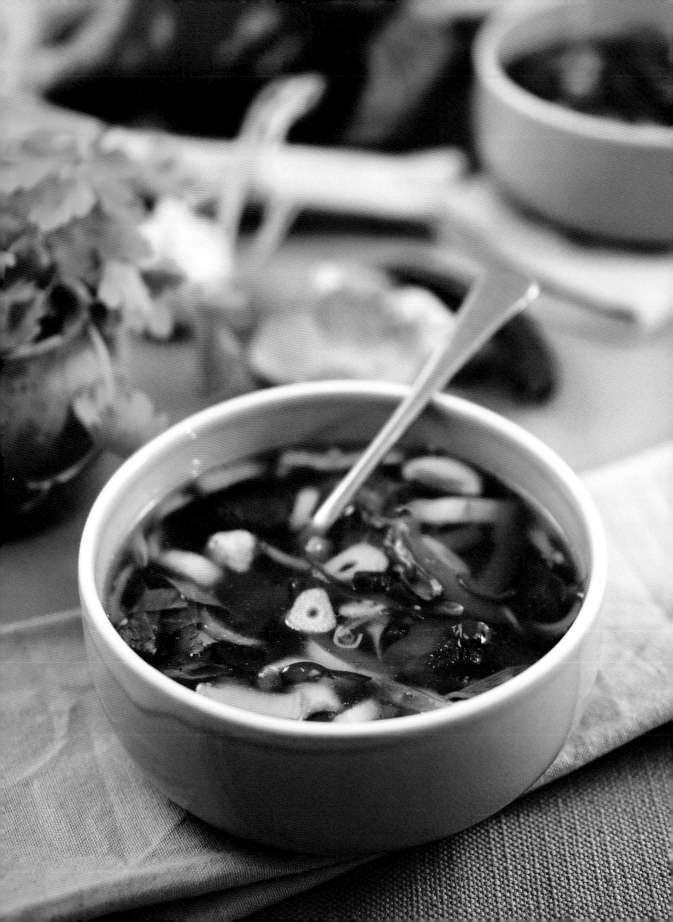

KATIE'S ORIENTAL SOUP......WITH A KICK

This is a clear soup and perfect for people who 'don't do soup' but love oriental food.
It is bursting with fresh, vibrant flavors and you can make a double batch of this soup and throw some rice noodles into the second batch, to make a Wagamama's style noodle soup. I'm personally not a fan of mushrooms, so I just pick these out, but Kate insists on keeping them in the recipe, as apparently shiitake mushrooms have a unique meaty texture and have been used by the Chinese for over 6 thousand years for their medicinal properties (and who am I to argue with that?!)

 GLUTEN-FREE

 VEGAN

 VEGETARIAN

INGREDIENTS:

Serves 2

Red Chillis
2 medium
Garlic
2 cloves
Ginger
approx. 20g or 2cm x 2cm chunk
Red Pepper
½ medium
Spring Onion
2 stalks
Bok Choi
1 bulb
Shiitake Mushrooms
50g or 4 medium
Fresh Coriander
10g or 1 small handful
Coconut Oil
1 tablespoon
Boiling Water
600 ml / 21 fl oz
Himalayan Rock Salt
1 pinch

PREPARE:

Preheat the oven to 160 °C (320 °F / gas mark 3).

Cut the chillis in half lengthways, remove the seeds, slice thinly and place half onto a baking tray. Peel the garlic and ginger. Remove the seeds from the red pepper. Remove the ends and outer skin from the spring onions. Remove the end from the bok choi. Thinly slice the garlic, ginger, spring onion, red pepper, bok choi and the mushrooms. Remove the leaves and discard the stems from the coriander.

COOK:

Put the chillis (on the baking tray) in the oven and cook for 2 minutes. Place the coconut oil in a pan and warm over a medium heat. Add the remaining chilli, garlic, ginger, spring onion, red pepper and mushrooms and cook for 5 minutes, stirring intermittently. Add the water and salt, reduce the heat and allow to simmer for 10 minutes, add the bok choi and coriander and simmer for a further 5 minutes.

SERVE:

Pour into your bowl of choice and sprinkle with the crispy chilli flakes.

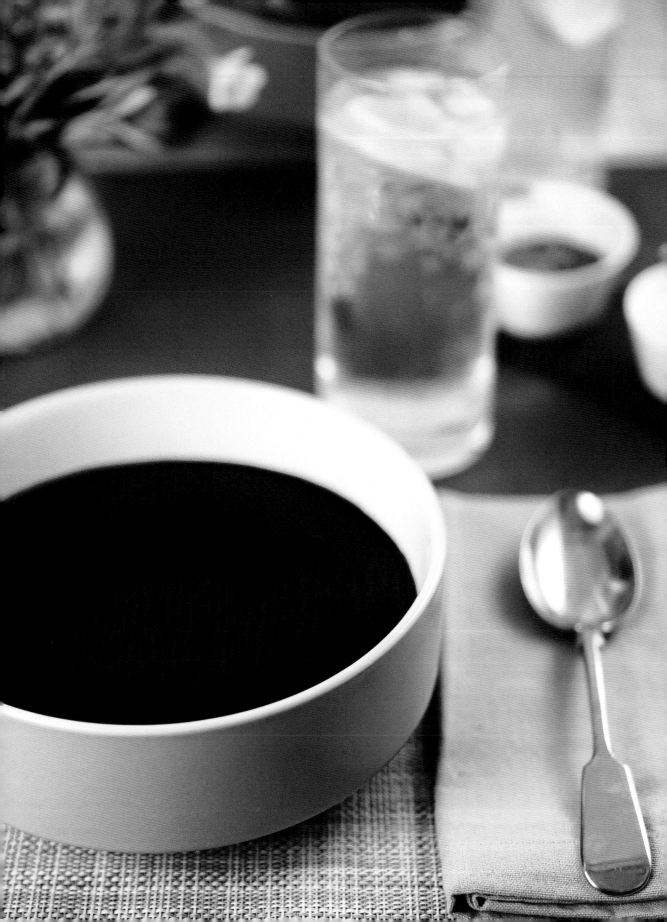

SWEET POTATO, BEETROOT & GINGER SOUP

GLUTEN-FREE

VEGAN

VEGETARIAN

This soup is wonderful at any time of year, but particularly special when the winter nights creep in. The sweet potato really gives it the hearty thick soup feel you want whilst the natural therapeutic root that is ginger provides a lovely kicker. Simple to make, oozing with nutrition and hits the mark on flavour. Sweet potato provides good amounts of vital minerals such as iron, calcium, magnesium, manganese and potassium that are very essential for enzyme, protein, and carbohydrate metabolism — and that's just the sweet potato. A true super soup, best served in front of an open fire in your PJ's!

INGREDIENTS:

Serves 2

Red Onion
1 small
Sweet Potato
1 medium
Beetroot (raw!)
1 medium bulb
Ginger
20g or 2cm x 2cm chunk
Olive Oil
1 tablespoon
Boiling Water
500 ml / 18 fl oz
Himalayan Rock Salt
1 pinch
Ground Black Pepper
1 generous pinch

PREPARE:

Remove the ends and skin from the onion and dice. Peel the sweet potato, remove any hard ends and chop into small chunks. Remove the top and any hard skin from the beetroot and chop into small chunks. Peel and chop the ginger into small pieces.

COOK:

Heat the olive oil in a pan over a medium heat, then add the red onion, sweet potato and beetroot, cover with a lid and cook for 10 minutes, stirring occasionally. Add the ginger and boiling water, reduce the heat and simmer for 10 minutes

BLEND:

Remove from the heat, add the salt and pepper and blend for 1 — 2 minutes, using a stick blender or regular upright blender. If using a regular blender **please be careful** as the steam creates pressure that can blow the lid off. Always cover the lid with a tea towel and hold down firmly whilst blending to avoid this.

SERVE:

In a beautiful bowl with a swirl of almond milk if you happen to have any already made in your fridge.

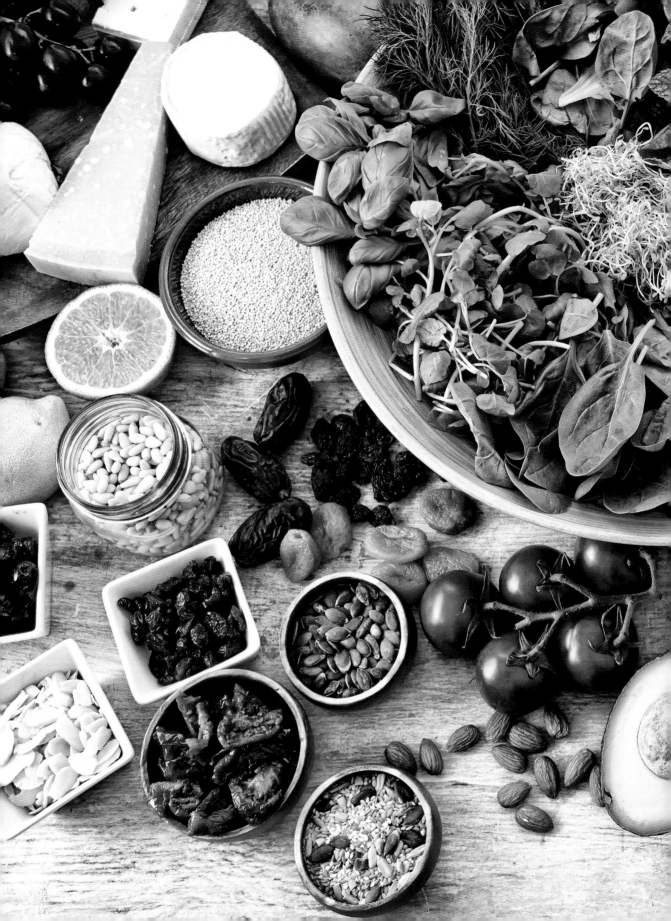

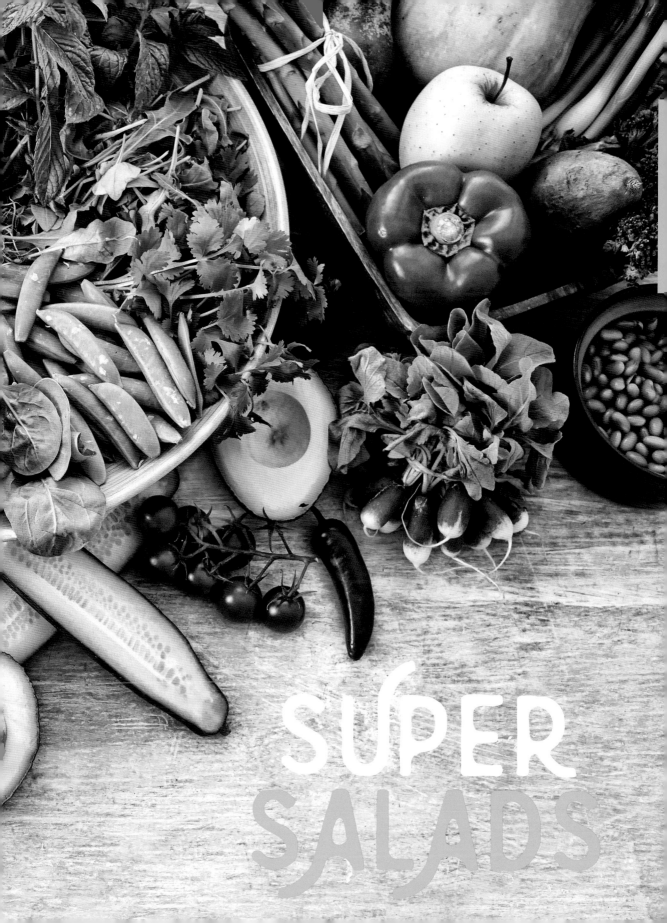

SUPER
SALADS

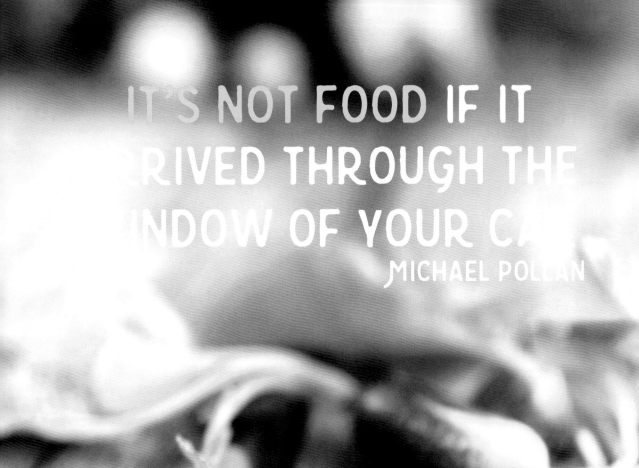

IT'S NOT FOOD IF IT
ARRIVED THROUGH THE
WINDOW OF YOUR CAR

MICHAEL POLLAN

NOT JUST FOR RABBITS!

I never thought in a million years I would ever even eat a salad, let alone write a cookbook with loads of my favorites in it! Salads, as far as I was concerned, were for rabbits and didn't represent what I considered to be real food. This was of course back in the days when I literally wouldn't eat anything that wasn't heavily processed and, if it even remotely resembled a leaf, it could go and take a running jump (like the rabbit itself!) The very idea of having only a salad for dinner was utterly ridiculous to me then. However, fast forward fifteen years and main course salads now make up a great deal of what I eat and my opinion that salads are 'only for rabbits' has been well and truly quashed.

I now LOVE a good main course salad and wonder how I survived for so many years without one! I say 'good' salad as some attempts at a main course salad can leave a great deal to be desired, even in some restaurants. A bit of dried cucumber and tomato on top of a load of iceberg lettuce really doesn't constitute a salad and it's no wonder many people feel a salad isn't really a meal, if that's their only experience of what one looks like.

The salads in this section are a beautiful eclectic mix of hot and cold, classic and new and they all, without exception, hit the buttons you'd want and expect them to.

In this Super Salad section, you'll find:

- ❋ WARM GOATS CHEESE SALAD WITH RED ONION MARMALADE (page 81)
- ❋ SUPER QUINOA SALAD...WITH A KICK! (page 99)
- ❋ WARM GINGER INFUSED BUTTERNUT SQUASH, PEAR & PARMESAN SALAD (page 101)
- ❋ SUPER GREEK-'ISH' SALAD (page 91)

All have something a little extra to give them that certain je ne sais quoi which transforms them from the black and white to full Technicolor so there's something in this section that is guaranteed to float your particular salad boat.

Remember to snap a pic of whichever super salad takes your fancy and share it on social media to spread the Super *fast* Food message and help to make a difference.

#superfastfood

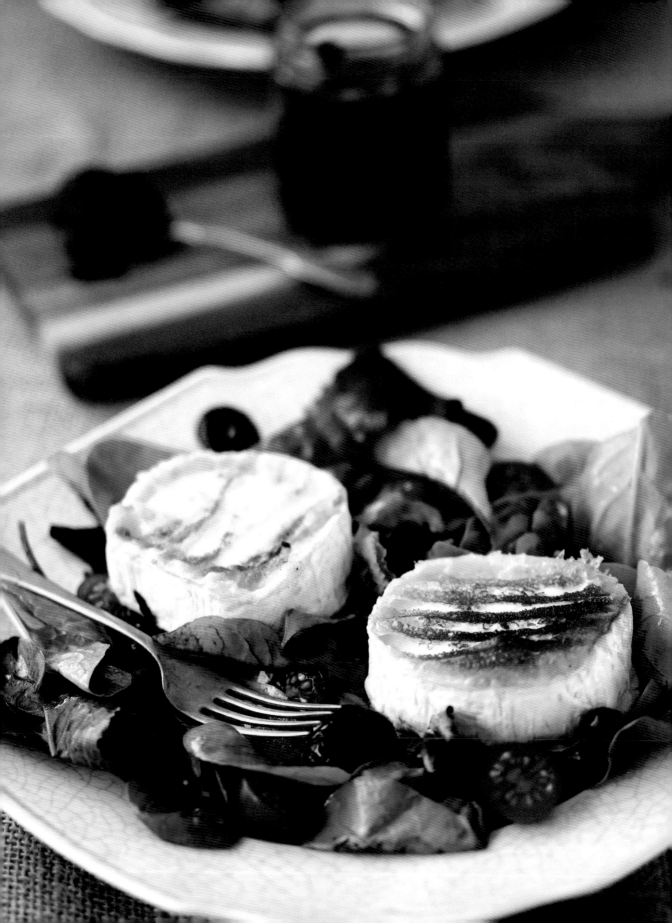

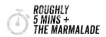

WARM GOATS CHEESE SALAD
WITH RED ONION MARMALADE

GLUTEN-FREE

VEGETARIAN

If you've ever been to my juice retreat in Portugal — Juicy Oasis — you may have already had the pleasure of enjoying this gorgeous salad. Although it's a 'juice only' retreat, on day seven you have the option of breaking your fast with a freshly made, nutritious salad and this particular one has been a firm favourite. The tang of the warm goats cheese is calmed beautifully by the red onion marmalade. The key behind getting the full impact of this dish, is to make sure you have a little of everything on your fork at the same time. Perfect as a main course with a cheeky side of sweet potato fries or equally good as a starter – just halve the ingredients. Hope you love this as much as I do!

INGREDIENTS:

Serves 2

Red Onion Marmalade
Page 113
Goats Cheese
400g/14oz
Cherry Tomatoes
8
Black Olives (pitted)
70g or 1 large handful
Mixed Leaves
100g or 2 large handfuls
Olive Oil
1 tablespoon
Balsamic Vinegar
1 teaspoon

PREPARE:

Firstly, make the Red Onion Marmalade – page 113.

Slice the goats cheese into pieces roughly 2 cm wide or 100g each. Chop the cherry tomatoes in half and place in a salad bowl along with the black olives and mixed leaves. Drizzle over the oil and vinegar and lightly mix.

COOK:

Place a dry griddle on the hob and turn the heat up nice and high. Once the griddle is hot, add the goats cheese and allow to sear for 1 – 2 minutes, before turning and repeating on the other side.

SERVE:

Pop the salad on your plate, place the goats cheese on top and finish with a generous spoonful of the red onion marmalade.

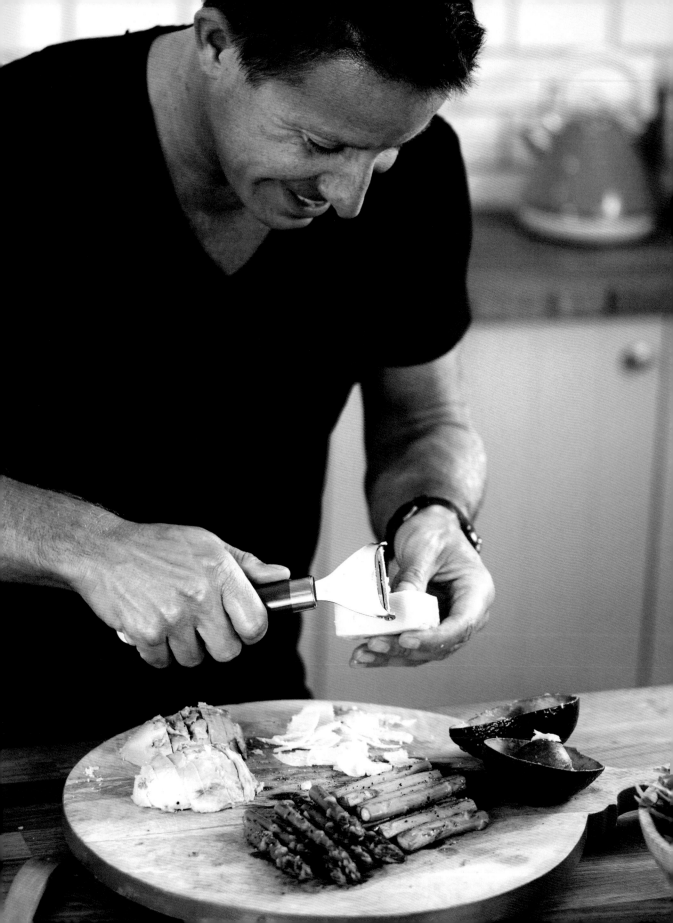

ROCKET, AVOCADO, GRILLED ASPARAGUS & SHAVED PARMESAN WITH A ROASTED GARLIC, LEMON & HONEY DRESSING

GLUTEN-FREE

VEGAN

VEGETARIAN

This simple salad contains the bad boys of the nutrition world — avocado, asparagus and garlic. Avocado is the single most nutritious stand-alone food in the world and garlic is known as 'Nature's Doctor' because of its antibiotic properties. Rocket leaves are a good source of vitamins A, C & K and minerals copper and iron. Asparagus has long been used in many traditional medicines to treat conditions like irritable bowel syndrome. It was of course Hippocrates who famously said 'Let Food Be Thy Medicine & Medicine Be Thy Food' and under its simple looking exterior, this superfood salad packs one hell of a nutritional punch. The Roasted Garlic, Lemon & Honey Dressing gives it the final taste finish that it needs to take it from 'okay' to 'out the park'.

SALAD INGREDIENTS:

Serves 2

Roasted Garlic, Lemon & Honey Dressing
Page 115

Asparagus Spears
8

Olive Oil
2 tablespoons

Ground Black Pepper
1 generous pinch

Avocado (ripe)
2 medium

Parmesan or Parmigiano Reggiano Cheese*
75g/3oz

Rocket
100g or 2 large handfuls

PREPARE:

Firstly, make the Roasted Garlic, Lemon & Honey Dressing page 115. Remove any hard ends from the asparagus, cut in half and place on a plate. Pour over half the olive oil, sprinkle with the black pepper, turning each piece so it is coated in the olive oil. Cut the avocados in half; remove the stones, scoop out the flesh and cut into generous slices. Shave the cheese with a vegetable peeler into very thin slices. Put the rocket into a bowl, drizzle over the remaining olive oil and lightly toss.

COOK:

Heat a griddle pan on a hot ring, add the asparagus and allow to cook for 2 — 3 minutes before turning and cooking for a further 2 – 3 minutes.

SERVE:

Place the rocket onto the middle of a plate, add the avocado, asparagus and cheese and drizzle over the dressing.

* If vegan leave these out

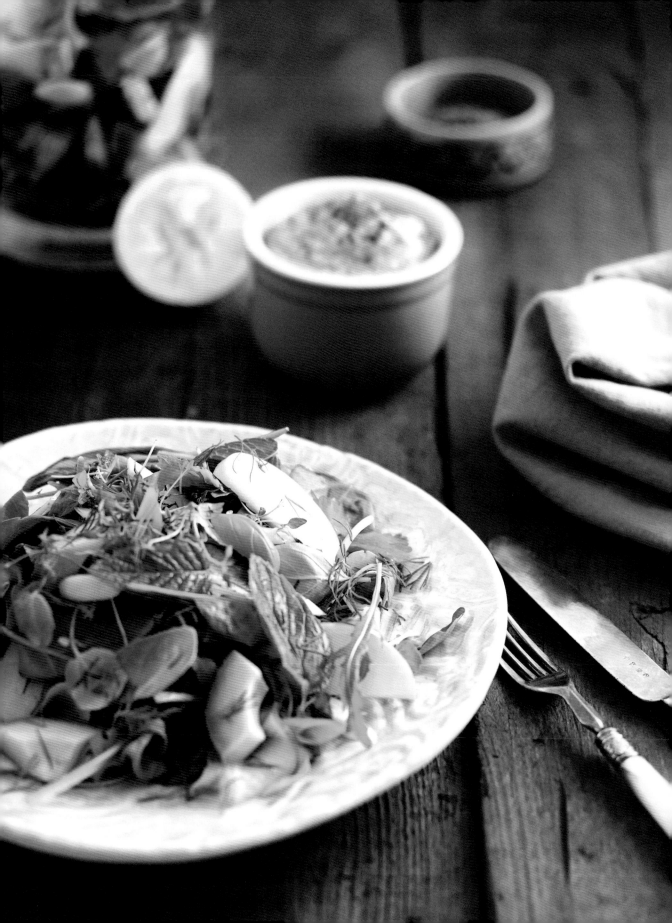

THE GREEN GODDESS SALAD WITH A SIDE OF MINT 'N' ROCKET HUMMUS

GLUTEN-FREE

VEGAN

VEGETARIAN

There's the hummus you buy in the shops, then there's the beautiful, creamy Mint 'N' Rocket Hummus you make fresh at home. It's this minty, zesty, yet simple side dish that transforms an already beautifully refreshing salad from 'oh that's nice' to 'OMG that's amazing!' It presses all the usual nutritional buttons – vitamins, minerals, phytonutrients, essential fats, amino acids etc. However something quite incredible happens when you combine all of the flavours of this dish together in one mouthful. The creaminess of the avocado is complimented beautifully by the hummus, whilst the herbs help to create a variety box of taste sensations with every forkful.

INGREDIENTS:

Serves 2

Mint 'N' Rocket Hummus
Page 239
Cucumber
½
Spring Onion
2 stalks
Green Apple
1
Avocado (ripe)
2 medium
Fresh Basil
25g or 1 small handful
Fresh Coriander
20g or 1 small handful
Fresh Mint
20g or 1 small handful
Fresh Dill
20g or 1 small handful
Fresh Thyme
20g or 1 small handful
Watercress
30g or 1 small handful
Baby Leaf Spinach
30g or 1 small handful
Rocket
30g or 1 small handful
Olive Oil
1 tablespoon
Ground Black Pepper
1 generous pinch
Lemon (the juice of)
½

PREPARE:

Firstly, make the Mint 'N' Rocket Hummus page 239.
Cut the cucumber in half, slice into thin slivers using a vegetable peeler, discarding any slices that are predominantly just skin. Remove the end and outer layer from the spring onion and slice into longish diagonal slices. Cut the apple into quarters; remove the core and slice thinly. Cut the avocados in half; remove the stone, scoop out the flesh and chop into chunks. Remove the leaves from the basil, coriander and mint and discard the stalks. Remove the hard stems from the dill and thyme and chop.

SERVE:

Place all the ingredients, except the hummus in a salad bowl, mix well then serve with a generous dollop of hummus.

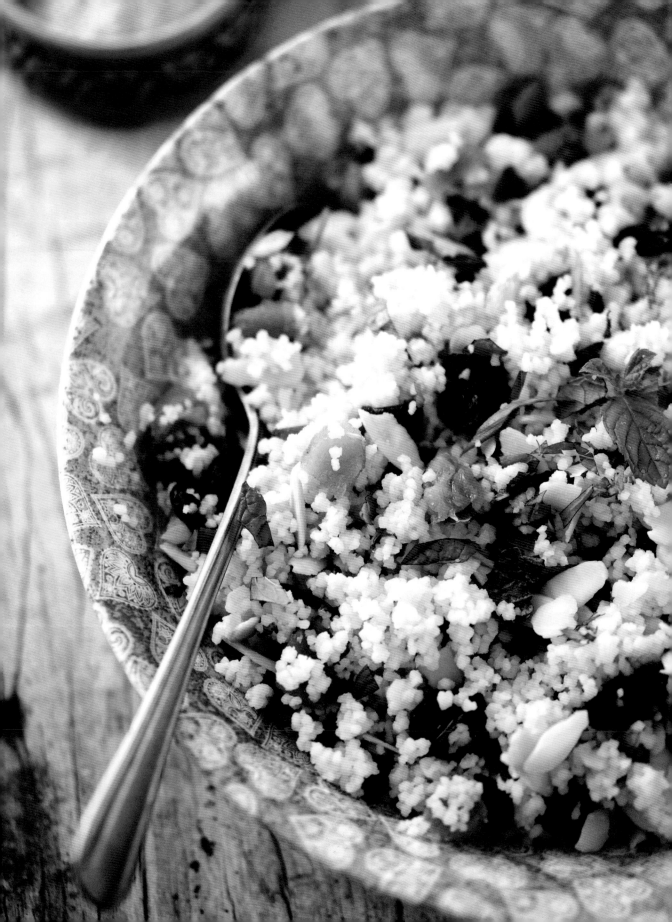

FRUITY COUSCOUS WITH ALMOND FLAKES & TAHINI, LEMON & MINT DRESSING

Not all salads have a lettuce leaf foundation and this fruity couscous salad is a shining example of a 'no lettuce' salad. What gives it that certain something which I feel all dishes of this nature require, is the Tahini, Lemon & Mint Dressing. Not only does this provide an excellent source of B vitamins and essential fatty acids, but it also transforms what could otherwise be a bland couscous salad into something exciting and full of flavour. OK so I am doing the stand-alone couscous salad a little disservice as it's actually pretty tasty on its own, but we're not looking for 'pretty tasty' we're looking for 'are you kidding me Vale!' when it comes to flavours. Healthy food of the past could be accused of being like cardboard and every recipe in this book has had to reach superfood status, whilst at the same time be 'dancing on your taste buds' tasty. This simple dish hits these requirements in abundance — enjoy!

INGREDIENTS:

Serves 2

Tahini, Lemon & Mint Dressing
Page 119

Spring Onion
1 stalk

Oranges
2 large

Apricots (un-sulphured
if possible)
6

Fresh Mint
20g or 1 small handful

Couscous
150g/5oz

Tap Water
Refer to instructions

Himalayan Rock Salt
1 pinch

Raisins
20g or 1 small handful

Cranberries (dried)
20g or 1 small handful

Almond Flakes
20g or 1 small handful

PREPARE:

Make the Tahini, Lemon & Mint dressing – page 119

Remove the end and the outer layer from the spring onion and slice thinly. Cut the oranges in half and squeeze the juice into a saucepan. Chop the apricots into pieces (similar size to a raisin). Remove the leaves from the mint, discard the stalks and chop finely. Rinse the couscous.

COOK:

Add enough water to the orange juice until you reach 225ml, then pour into a saucepan along with the salt and couscous. Bring to the boil and then reduce the heat and simmer for 5 minutes, stirring sporadically and keeping a watchful eye on the liquid. As soon as it has all absorbed, remove from the heat.

COMBINE:

Allow the couscous to stand for about 10 minutes and then add the raisins, cranberries, apricots, almonds, spring onion, mint, dressing and mix well.

SERVE:

Enjoy slightly warm or allow to cool, the choice is yours!

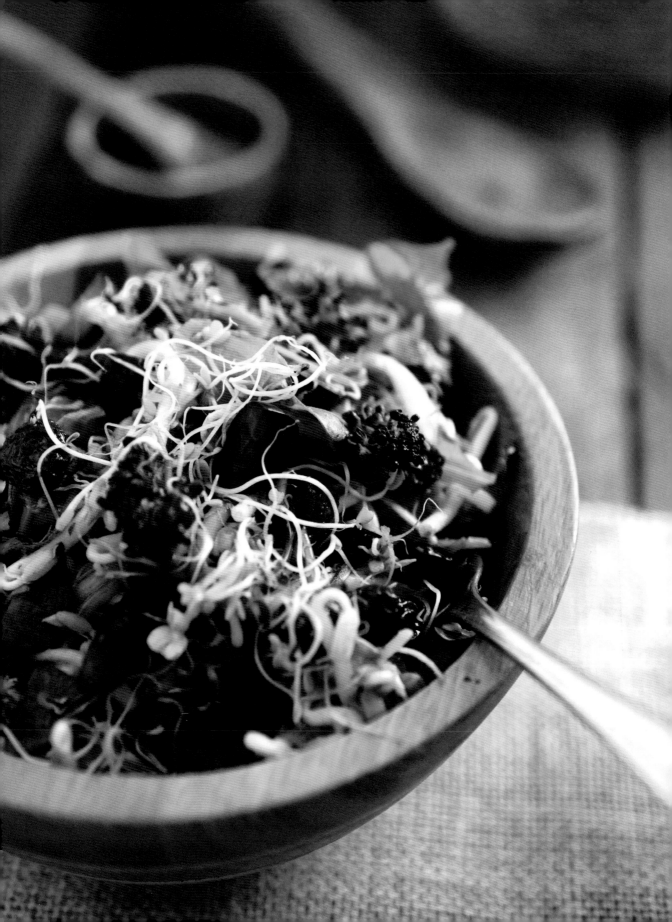

SUPER SPROUTING SALAD WITH A GINGER, CHILLI & SESAME DRESSING

The good news is, with superfoods finally coming into the everyday life and consciousness of the majority, we can finally get our hands on what were, in the past, considered 'obscure' ingredients, pretty much anywhere — including most major supermarkets. Sprouts are one such ingredient which we no longer have to go to some random independent health food store down the back street of nowhere to get. 'Live' sprouts are arguably one of the worlds top superfoods and this, therefore, could be argued as being one of the most nutritious salads in this book. The list of vitamins, minerals and other phytonutrients contained in this salad is simply too long to fit into this space. However, name any vitamin or mineral and chances are it will be working its magic somewhere in this light and tasty dish. Perfect for al fresco dining on a beautiful summers day, as vitamin D is perhaps the only vitamin nutrient missing from the dish itself.

INGREDIENTS:

Serves 2

Ginger, Chilli & Sesame Dressing
Page 117

Purple Sprouting Broccoli
100g/3.5oz

Red Grapes (seedless)
100g or 1 handful

Sprouted Alfalfa
25g or 1 small handful

Clover Sprouts (or similar)
25g or 1 small handful

Broccoli Sprouts (or similar)
25g or 1 small handful

Radish Sprouts (or similar)
25g or 1 small handful

Bean Sprouts
100g or 1 large handful

Raisins
70g or 1 handful

Rocket
50g or 1 handful

PREPARE:

Make the Ginger, Chilli & Sesame Dressing — page 117

Remove the florets from the broccoli (save the stalks for tomorrow's juice) and break into small pieces. Cut the grapes in quarters. Add all the ingredients and the dressing to a mixing bowl and combine.

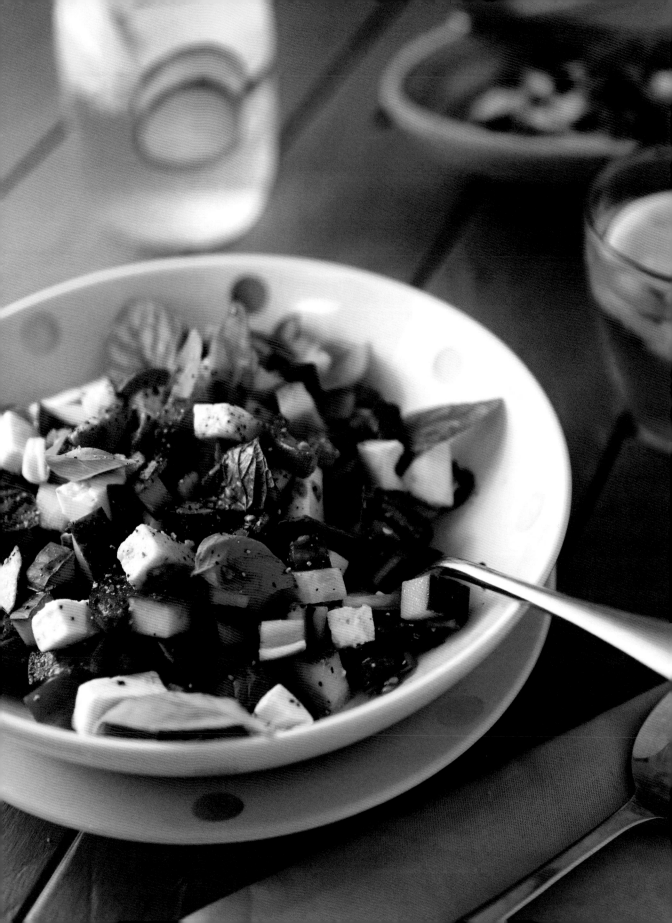

SUPER GREEK-'ISH' SALAD

GLUTEN-FREE

VEGETARIAN

Greek Salad is one of those classic salads that you simply cannot leave out of any superfood recipe book. It could be argued that 'if it aint broke then don't try to fix it' but I believe everything can be improved upon, even this classic. The good news is I haven't gone too far off course and it's still very much 'Greek', but with a nice twist. That twist comes in the form of fresh mint and basil. These two seemingly innocuous nutritious herbs just add the lift I have always felt the classic Greek Salad needed. If I'm honest, I personally also leave out the raw onion when I make this as I hate raw onion, but I was vetoed from leaving it out of this version. As always the Greek-'ish' Salad is the perfect light, main course lunch but works extremely well as starter too — just halve the ingredients.

INGREDIENTS:

Serves 2

Lemon (the juice of)
½

Olive Oil
1 tablespoon

Fresh Mint
20g or 1 small handful

Fresh Basil
20g or 1 small handful

Red Onion (small)
½

Tomatoes (medium)
4

Cucumber
½

Feta Cheese
150g/5oz

Black Olives (pitted)
70g or 1 handful

Himalayan Rock Salt
1 pinch

Ground Black Pepper
1 generous pinch

PREPARE:

In a small bowl, combine the lemon juice with the olive oil.

Remove the mint and basil leaves and discard the stalks. Remove the ends from the onion and peel. Cut the tomatoes, cucumber, feta and onion into lovely small pieces.

SERVE:

Place all the ingredients in a salad bowl; add the lemon and oil, salt and pepper and mix.

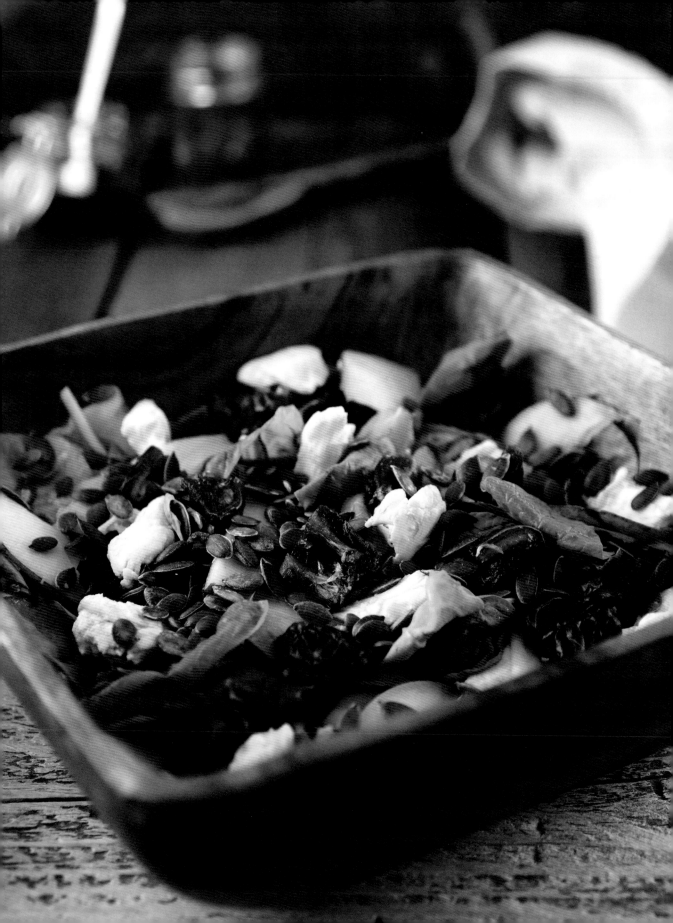

MOZZARELLA, PEAR & DATE SALAD, DRIZZLED WITH AN ORANGE & BALSAMIC REDUCTION

GLUTEN-FREE

VEGETARIAN

I was a vegan for many years and the one thing I missed more than anything else was cheese. I like most cheeses but there's something about mozzarella that makes it stand out from the cheesy crowd. You may immediately think that the fact it's made from buffalo and not cow's milk is the clear defining deference, but mozzarella is often made from cow's milk too. No, the defining factor is its moisture content and texture. Most cheeses are chewy but mozzarella is what I describe as the 'oyster' of the cheese world as it tends to just slide down the throat. The combination of pear, dates and this beautiful cheese is one to cherish. Add the sweet and tangy Orange & Balsamic Reduction and you take this already beautiful combination to a level of decadence rarely seen outside of Mayfair.

INGREDIENTS:

Serves 2

Orange & Balsamic Reduction
Page 115
Pear (ripe)
1
Dates (Medjool are the best)
6
Mozzarella
240g/8.5oz
Mixed Leaves
120g or 2 large handfuls
Pumpkin Seeds
30g or 1 small handful

PREPARE:

Make the Orange & Balsamic Reduction — page 115

Cut the pear into quarters, remove the core and thinly slice.
Remove any hard ends and stones from the dates and cut into quarters.
Tear the mozzarella into bite sized chunks (it looks better than when cut with a knife).

SERVE:

Place the pear, dates, mozzarella, mixed leaves, pumpkin seeds and the balamic reduction into a salad bowl and toss.

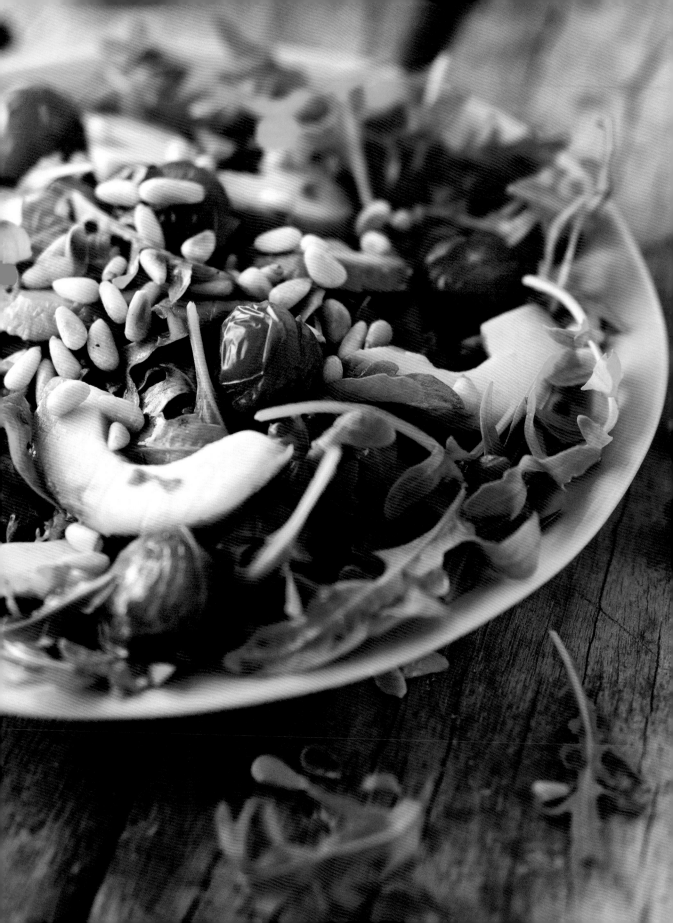

AVOCADO & ROCKET WITH ROASTED CHERRY TOMATOES, TOASTED PINE NUTS & LEMON PESTO DRESSING

GLUTEN-FREE

VEGETARIAN

CONTAINS NUTS

As a main course salad it's hard to top this. Avocado and rocket were always destined to be together, but were always going to be far too 'vanilla' in any relationship on their own. By adding roasted cherry tomatoes, toasted pine nuts and a lemon pesto dressing to die for, you bring these two magnificent superfoods out of the 'Monday morning' and straight into the 'Saturday night'! The texture, flavour and sheer level of genuine natural nutrients, makes this one of the salads you'll come to time and time again. It's stupidly easy to make and is spot on in terms of the Super *fast* Food title of the book. Although beautiful as a main on its own, a few cheeky sweet potato wedges on the side never did anyone any harm.

INGREDIENTS:

Serves 2

Lemon Pesto Dressing
Page 113

Cherry Tomatoes
12

Avocado (ripe)
2 medium

Pine Nuts
50g or 1 handful

Rocket
120g or 2 large handfuls

Olive Oil
1 tablespoon

PREPARE:

Preheat the grill to a high heat

Prepare the Lemon Pesto Dressing – page 113

Remove the stalks from the cherry tomato and place on a baking tray. Chop the avocados in half, discard the stone, remove the flesh and cut into good-sized slices.

COOK:

Place the baking tray under the grill and cook for 3 – 5 minutes, until the tomatoes start to brown slightly. Put the pine nuts into a frying pan (with no oil) and place on the hob over a medium to high heat for 2 – 3 minutes, turning constantly, until brown.

SERVE:

Place the rocket into a salad bowl, drizzle with the olive oil and toss. Add the avocado, tomatoes and pine nuts and drizzle with the lemon pesto dressing.

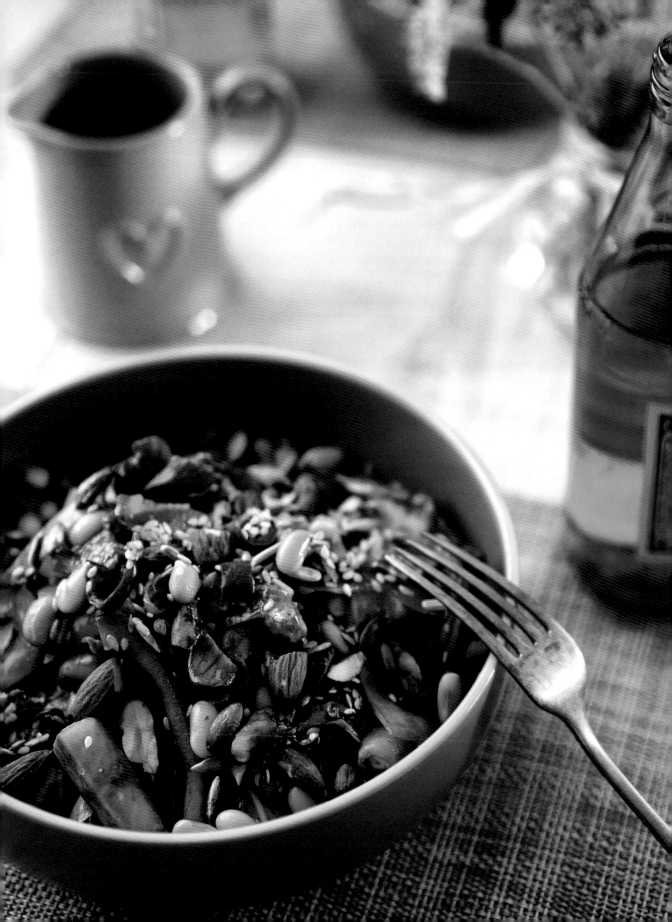

GLUTEN-FREE

 VEGAN

 VEGETARIAN

 CONTAINS NUTS

CRUNCHY MUNCHIE SALAD WITH A LIME, CHILLI & CORIANDER DRESSING

As the name suggests, this is one salad you can really get your teeth into and your body will be thankful you did. Loaded with vitamins A, B, C, E, and K as well as magnesium, iron, calcium and manganese, this snappy salad is also brimming with phytonutrients proven to have anti-inflammatory properties. Like all the recipes in this book — No Chef Required and hopefully after a few more meals like this one, no doctor required either!

INGREDIENTS:

Serves 2

Lime Chilli & Coriander Dressing
Page 117

Red Pepper
1 medium

Cucumber
¼ medium

Baby Leaf Spinach
60g or 1 large handful

Sugar Snap Peas
40g or 1 handful

Red Chilli
1 medium

Almonds (whole)
50g or 1 handful

Mixed Seeds
60g or 1 large handful

Himalayan Rock Salt
1 generous pinch

Fresh Edamame Beans
100g/3.5oz

PREPARE:

Lime Chilli & Coriander Dressing — page 117.

Preheat the oven to 180 °C (350 °F/ gas mark 4).

Finely slice the red pepper, removing the seeds and core. Using a vegetable peeler, slice the cucumber lengthways to create very thin strips (discarding any slices that are just skin). Chop the spinach. Remove the ends from the sugar snap peas and any stringy bits from the spine, and then cut in half. Remove the top from the chilli, cut in half, remove the seeds, and slice finely. Coarsely chop the almonds and place on a backing tray along with the chilli, mixed seeds and the salt.

HEAT:

Place the baking tray in the oven and cook for 5 minutes

COMBINE:

Put all the ingredients, along with the dressing into a salad bowl and mix thoroughly.

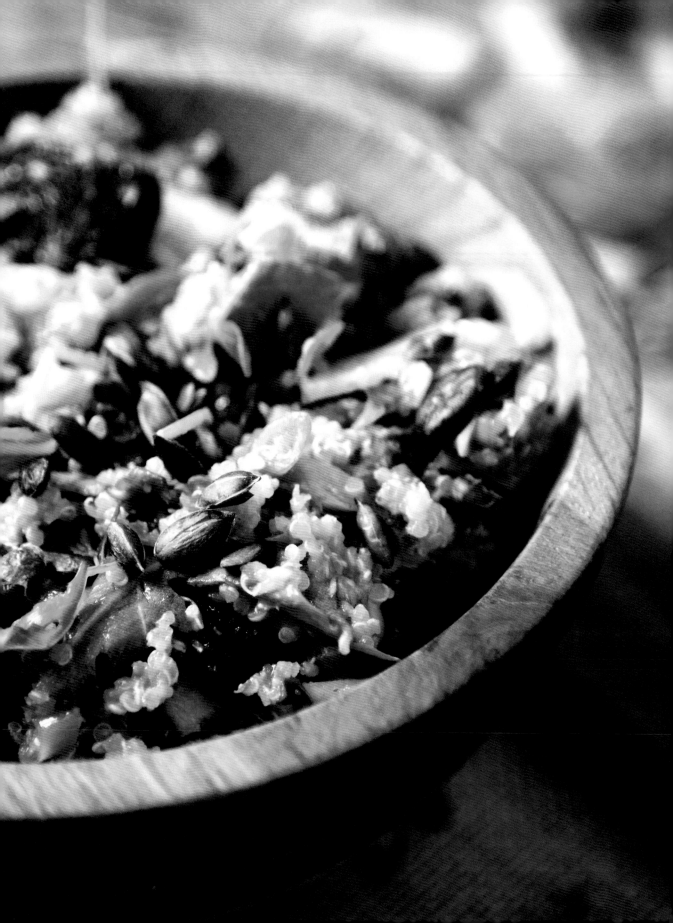

SUPER QUINOA SALAD...WITH A KICK!

GLUTEN-FREE

VEGAN

VEGETARIAN

Quinoa is the new 'grain kid' on the block and it seems to have knocked the traditional grain 'kings', such as rice, off the top of the 'healthy carb' charts. Hard to pronounce ('keen-wa') but easy to digest, quinoa has twice the protein content of rice or barley and is also a very good source of calcium, magnesium and manganese. It also possesses good levels of several B vitamins, vitamin E and that all important dietary fibre. On its own I find this grain pretty bland, and whatever you combine with it, you'll always find it needs a kick of some kind. The kick here comes from the Dijon mustard dressing, the spring onion and of course those cheeky little sun-blushed tomatoes. Rich in amino acids, fatty acids, vitamins, minerals and a plethora of phytonutrients, all of which help it to superfood status.

INGREDIENTS:

Serves 2

Quinoa
100g/3.5oz
Cold Tap Water
300ml/11fl oz
Pumpkin Seeds
45g or 1 large handful
Himalayan Rock Salt
1 pinch
Spring Onion
2 stalks
Cucumber
¼
Sun-Blushed Tomatoes
100g/3.5oz
Rocket
40g or 1 handful

INGREDIENTS FOR THE DRESSING:

Lemon (the juice of)
1
Olive Oil
100ml/3.5fl oz
Honey*
2 heaped teaspoons
Dijon Mustard
2 level teaspoons

PREPARE:

Wash and drain the quinoa and place in a pan with the cold water.

COOK:

Place the pan on the hob and bring to boil, then reduce the heat, cover with a lid and allow to simmer for 15 – 20 minutes until all the liquid has been absorbed. Keep a beady eye on the quinoa, so that at the stage when all the water has evaporated you can remove it from the heat, transfer into a large bowl and allow to cool.

MEANWHILE LET'S TOAST:

Place the pumpkin seeds and salt in a dry frying pan and pop over a high heat for 2 — 5 minutes until they start to brown, then remove and allow to cool.

MAKE THE DRESSING:

Place all the ingredients for the dressing into an old jar and shake well until all are combined.

PREPARE:

Remove the end and outer skin from the spring onion and slice finely. Slice the cucumber and then chop each slice into quarters. Chop the sun-blushed tomatoes.

SERVE:

Combine everything together including the dressing and mix well.

* If vegan please use an alternative sweetener.

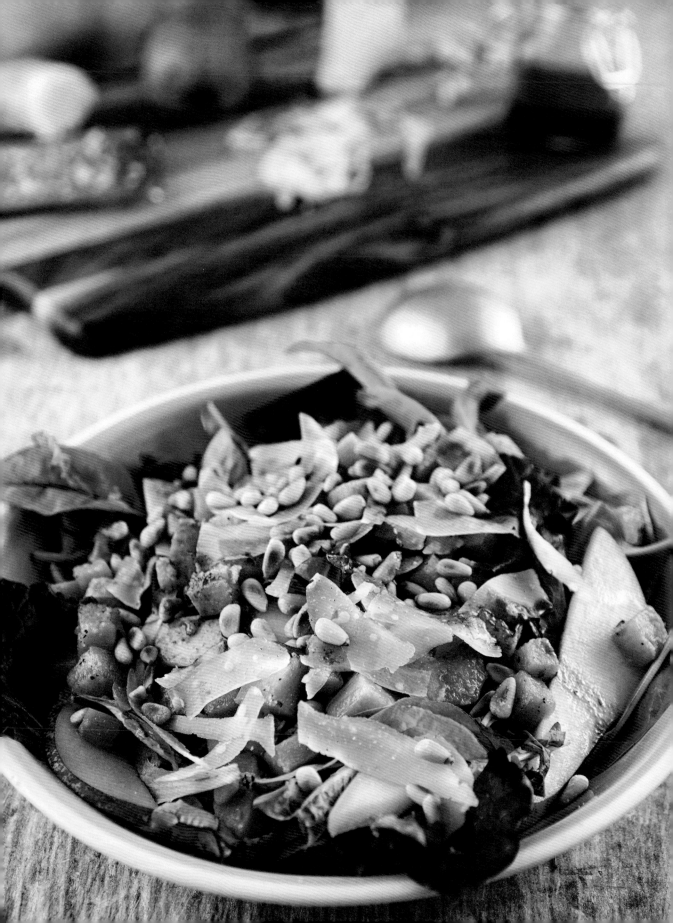

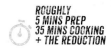

WARM GINGER INFUSED BUTTERNUT SQUASH, PEAR & PARMESAN SALAD

Whoever said salads aren't for winter has never tasted this baby! The second you add any warmth to a salad I feel you totally transform it, from something light to have for lunch on a fine summers day, to a genuinely warming meal that can be enjoyed anytime. The ginger infused butternut squash and toasted pine nuts are the real stars here. Packed with an abundance of nutrition and flavor, this dish is also unbelievably filling. Unlike a lot of salads, where I'm often tempted to have a nice cheeky side of sweet potato fries, I find I need nothing extra to satisfy my appetite when having this.

GLUTEN-FREE

VEGETARIAN

CONTAINS NUTS

INGREDIENTS:

Serves 2

Orange, & Balsamic
Reduction
Page 115

Butternut Squash
½ small

Olive Oil
2 tablespoon

Himalayan Rock Salt
1 pinch

Ground Black Pepper
1 generous pinch

Fresh Ginger
40g or 4 cm x 4 cm chunk

Pear (ripe)
1

Parmesan or Parmigiano Reggiano
Cheese
75g/3oz

Mixed Leaves
75g or 2 handfuls

Pine Nuts
50g or 1 handful

PREPARE:

Firstly, prepare the Orange & Balsamic Reduction page 115.

Preheat the oven to 180 °C (350 °F/gas mark 4).

Remove the ends from the butternut squash and peel. Cut in half, remove the seeds and chop into bite sized chunks (about 1 cm x 1 cm), then scatter onto a baking tray. Drizzle over half the oil and sprinkle over the salt and pepper. Peel, then grate the ginger directly onto the butternut squash and mix so that the squash is coated in oil and seasoning.

COOK:

Place the tray in the oven for 30 – 35 minutes until the squash is cooked.

MEANWHILE PREPARE:

Cut the pear into quarters; remove the core and slice into thin strips. Shave the cheese with a vegetable peeler into very thin slivers. Put the mixed leaves into a salad bowl; add the pear, remaining olive oil and lightly toss.

WARM:

When the butternut squash is cooked, remove from the oven. Heat a dry frying pan on the hob and toast the pine nuts for 2 – 3 minutes over a medium heat until golden, stirring continually, to avoid burning!

SERVE:

Put the salad leaves and pear onto a plate; add the butternut squash, cheese and pine nuts. Finish with a generous drizzle of the balsamic reduction.

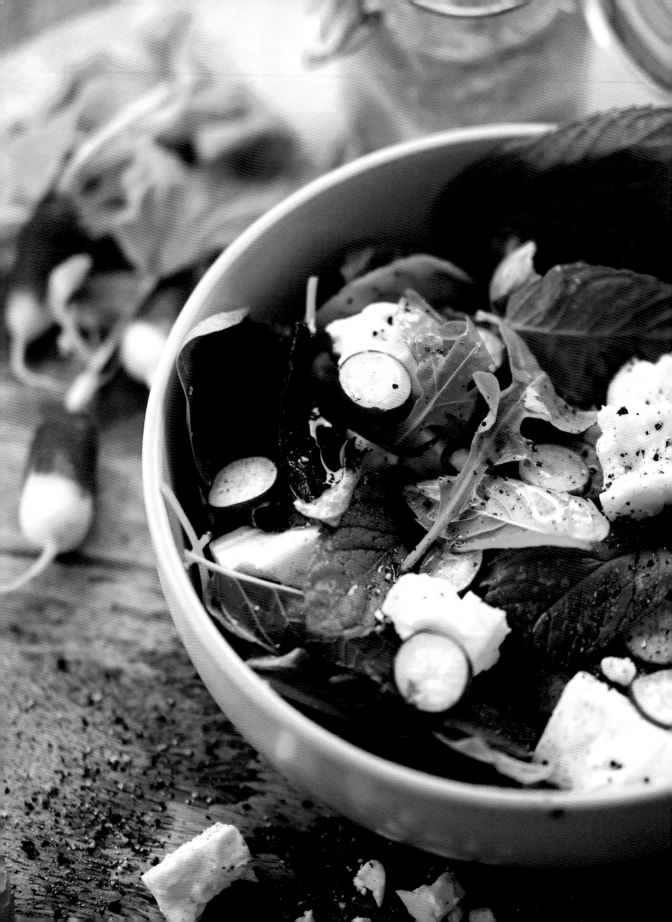

FETA & MINT SALAD WITH SHAVED RADISH & A ROASTED GARLIC, LEMON & HONEY DRESSING

GLUTEN-FREE

VEGETARIAN

CONTAINS NUTS

There's something about the beautiful combo of fresh mint and feta cheese that never fails to satisfy on every level. However, add the peppery flavors of some fresh radish, a few green leaves and a cheeky drizzle of sweet Roasted Garlic, Honey & Lemon Dressing and you have one hell of a fresh and nutrient rich dish. Garlic is known by many as the 'DR' of the food world and it could be argued there's no other food in the superfood charts higher than garlic. This Dr. Garlic, along with the radish and mint, help to make this salad a wonderful anti-inflammatory Super Salad. Enjoy!

INGREDIENTS:

Serves 2

Roasted Garlic, Lemon & Honey Dressing
Page 115

Feta Cheese
200g/7oz

Radishes
6

Fresh Mint
30g or 1 small handful

Mixed Leaves
100g or 2 large handfuls

Ground Black Pepper
1 generous pinch

PREPARE:

Make the Roasted Garlic, Lemon & Honey Dressing — page 115

Break the feta into bite sized pieces (about 1 cm x 1 cm).
Remove the ends from the radish' and slice very thinly with a sharp knife or vegetable peeler. Remove the leaves from the mint and discard the stems.

SERVE:

Place the radishes, mint and mixed leaves in a mixing bowl, pour over half the dressing and mix, then add the feta cheese, drizzle with the remaining dressing and finish off with the black pepper.

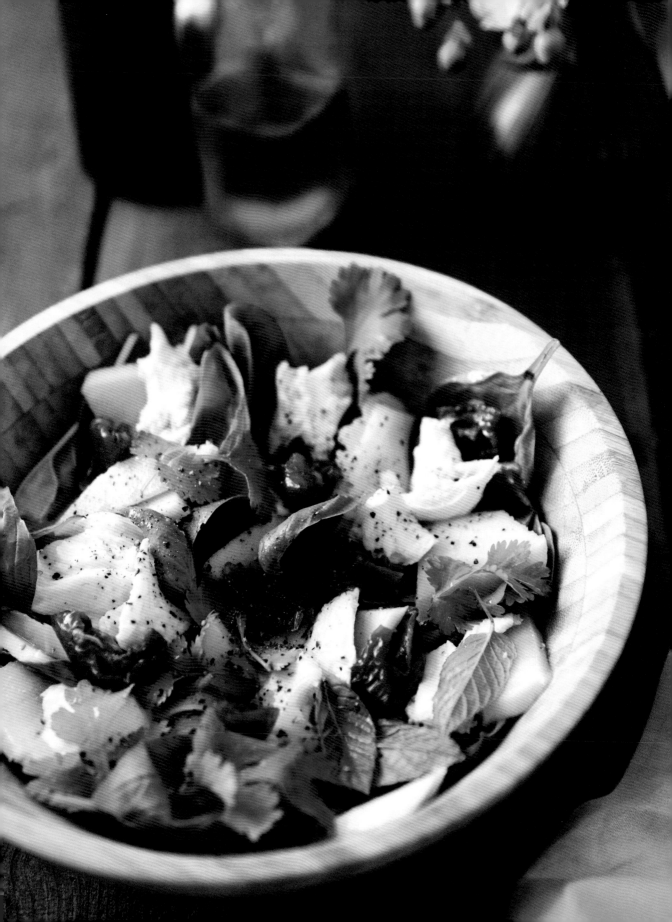

MOZZARELLA, MANGO & SUN-BLUSHED TOMATO ON A BED OF FRESH HERBS

I'm genuinely salivating just writing the description for this simple, yet 'out the park', Super Salad. Every ingredient seems to have been destined to come together in order to help create this exceptionally tasty and nutritious dish. The mozzarella, mango and sun-blushed tomatoes, combined with the fresh herbs, creates a spectrum of flavors that make you want to savour every single mouthful. There are many solid health reasons to have this salad, but you may like to know that mango has aphrodisiac properties and is known as the 'love fruit'. They have been said to increase the virility in men and are also loaded with vitamin E, which helps to regulate sex hormones and boosts sex drive, so enjoy!

INGREDIENTS:

Serves 2

Mango (ripe)
½
Fresh Basil
20g or 1 small handful
Fresh Mint
20g or 1 small handful
Fresh Coriander
20g or 1 small handful
Mozzarella
150g/5oz
Baby Leaf Spinach
40g or 1 handful
Sun-Blushed Tomatoes
60g/2oz
Olive Oil
1 tablespoon
Apple Cider Vinegar
1 teaspoon
Ground Black Pepper
1 generous pinch

PREPARE:

Remove the flesh from the mango, discard the skin and stone, then cut into slices. Remove the leaves from the basil, mint and coriander and discard the stalks. Tear the mozzarella into bite sized chunks (this looks so much better than when you cut it with a knife).

SERVE:

Place all the ingredients in a salad bowl, drizzle with the oil and vinegar, toss lightly and finish with a generous sprinkling of black pepper.

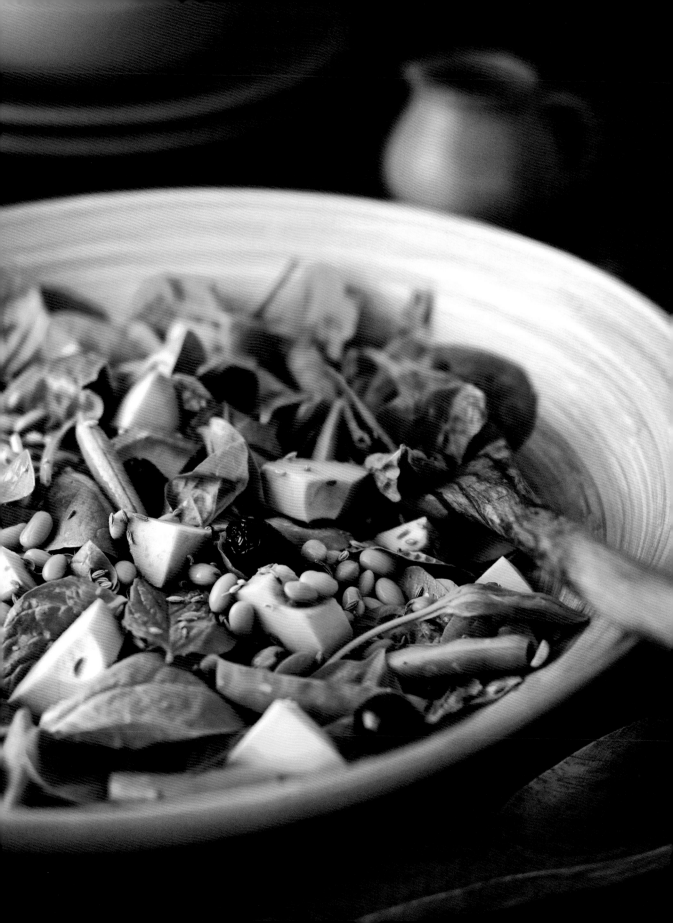

AVOCADO, MINT, FENNEL & EDAMAME SALAD WITH A GINGER, HONEY & YOGURT SPLASH

GLUTEN-FREE

VEGETARIAN

For me, avocado is the world's number one superfood. It's so rich, so creamy and yet mind-blowingly nutritious that it should be a staple in everyone's diet. In fact the avocado alone brings to the table in excess of 25 essential nutrients including vitamins A, B, C, E, K, copper, iron, phosphorous magnesium and potassium. The addition of fresh mint, fennel, ginger and honey takes this already delicious dish to a fragrant new level, where your taste buds and body will forever wish to remain!

INGREDIENTS:

Serves 2

Ginger, Honey & Yogurt Splash
Page 119

Avocado (ripe)
1 large

Sugar Snap Peas or Mange Tout
60g or 1 handful

Fresh Mint
20g or 1 small handful

Baby Leaf Spinach
100g or 2 large handfuls

Olive Oil
1 tablespoon

Fennel Seeds
1 tablespoon

Olives (pitted)
70g or 1 large handful

Edamame Beans
60g or 1 handful

PREPARE:

Make the Ginger, Honey & Yogurt Splash — page 119.

Cut the avocado in half, remove the stone, scoop out the flesh and cut into nice large chunks. Remove the ends and the stringy spines from the sugar snap peas/mange tout. Remove the leaves from the mint and discard the stalks.

COMBINE:

Put the mint, spinach and sugar snap peas/mange tout into a bowl, along with the olive oil and fennel seeds and mix. Place the salad onto the plates and add the avocado, olives and edamame beans, then drizzle with the dressing.

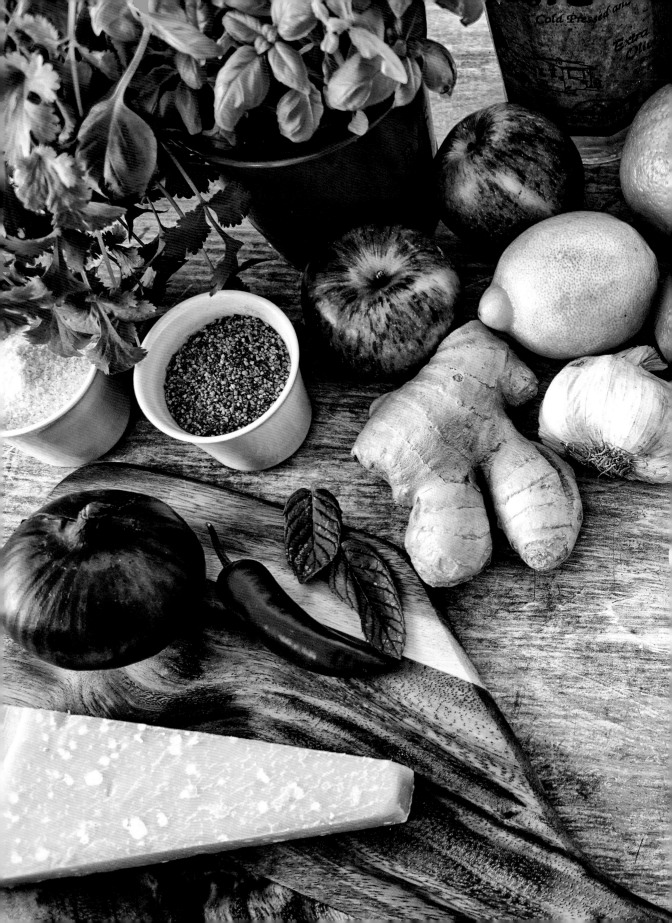

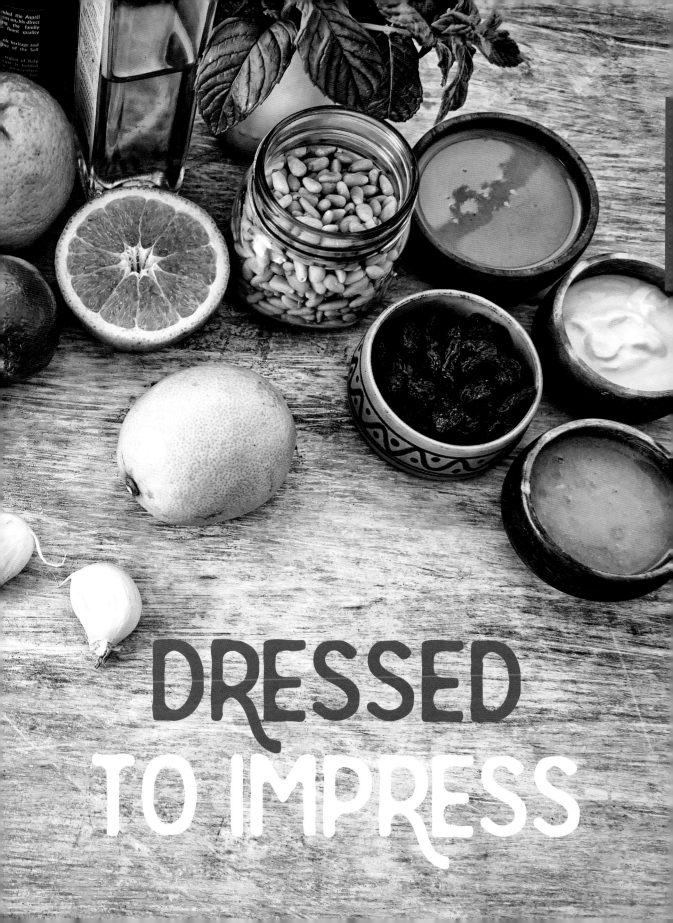

DRESSED
TO IMPRESS

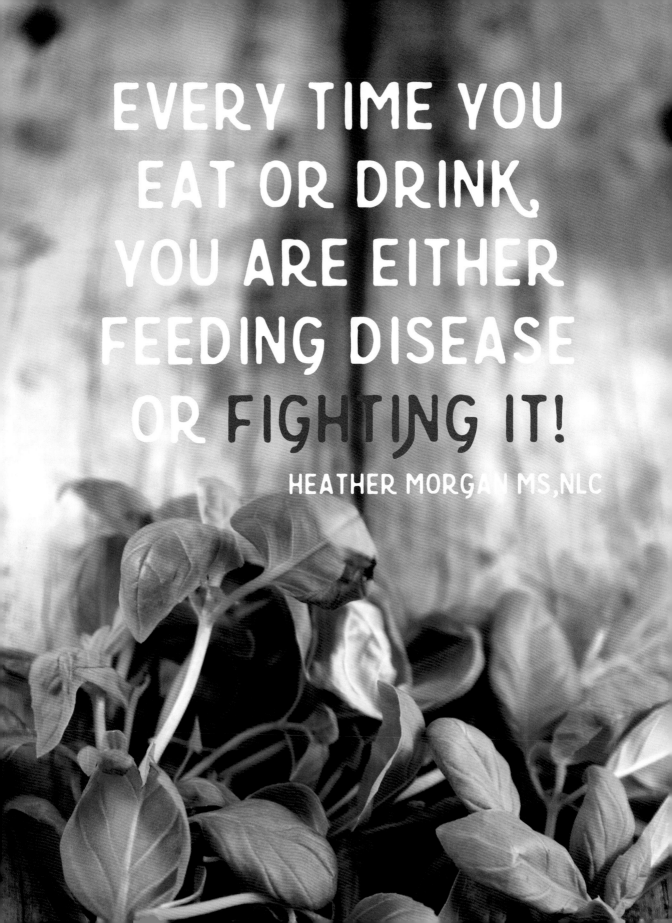

IT'S NOT ALWAYS WHAT'S UNDERNEATH THAT COUNTS!

Many dishes simply wouldn't be the same without being **Dressed to Impress** and the simple dressings you'll find in this section have the ability not only to enhance a dish, but to *make* a dish. Take the **Red Onion Marmalade** (page 113) for example, it completely transforms an otherwise regular warm goats cheese salad into something pretty special. If you have been to any of my retreats and have tasted the delights of the **Warm Goats Cheese Salad with Red Onion Marmalade** (page 81) at the end of the seven days of juicing, you'll already be aware of just how exceptionally good it is. Then you have something like the extremely easy to make **Lemon Pesto Dressing** (see page 113), that can take an otherwise bland green salad to another dimension. The point is, the final drizzle of a dressing can often be the je ne sais quoi that takes a dish to another level.

Here you'll find the ones I use the most:

- **RED ONION MARMALADE** (page 113)
- **LEMON PESTO DRESSING** (page 113)
- **ORANGE & BALSAMIC REDUCTION** (page 115)
- **ROASTED GARLIC, LEMON & HONEY DRESSING** (page 115)
- **LIME, CHILLI & CORIANDER DRESSING** (page 117)
- **GINGER, CHILLI & SESAME DRESSING** (page 117)
- **TAHINI, LEMON & MINT DRESSING** (page 119)
- **GINGER, HONEY & YOGURT SPLASH** (page 119)

You will find throughout the book I recommend a certain dressing to go along with a particular dish, but clearly dressings are often interchangeable and work well with a number of different dishes. Hope you love them and you'll find out that sometimes it's what's on top that counts!

Remember to snap a pic of whichever delightful dressing takes your fancy and share it on social media to spread the **Super *fast* Food** message and help to make a difference.

#superfastfood

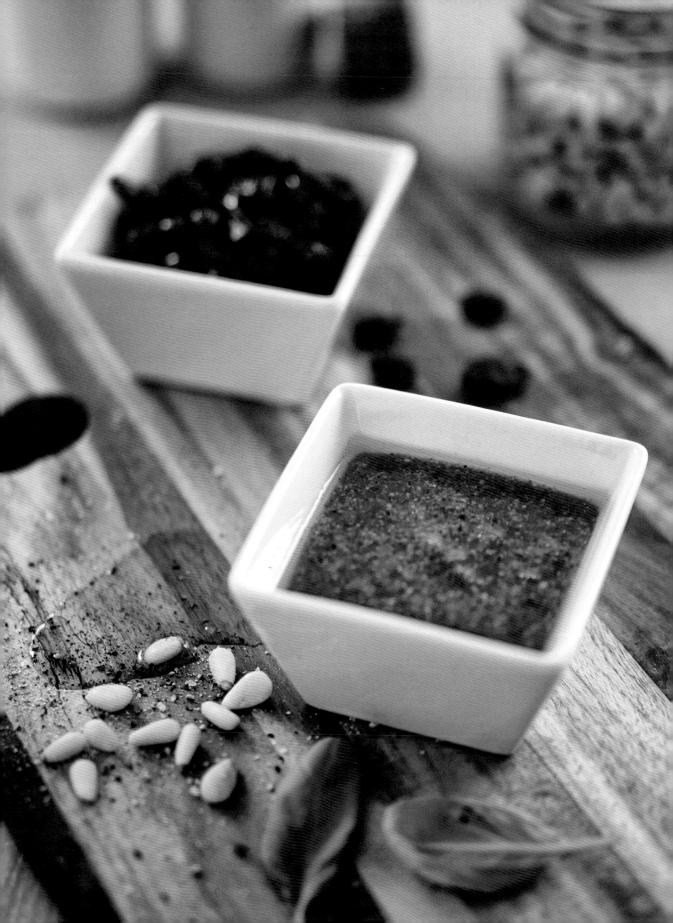

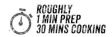

RED ONION MARMALADE

This genuinely stupidly delicious dressing goes with almost anything, but something magical happens when you add it to warm goats cheese. I personally hate raw onions; yet adore this warm, red onion marmalade. Hope it hits the spot for you too!

GLUTEN-FREE

VEGAN

VEGETARIAN

INGREDIENTS:

Serves 2

Red Onion (small)
1
Olive Oil
1 tablespoon
Apple Juice (ideally freshly extracted)
2 apples (if not 200ml/7fl oz)
Raisins
30g or 1 handful
Balsamic Vinegar
2 tablespoons

PREPARE:

Remove the ends from the onion, peel, cut in half and slice into thin slices.

COOK:

Drizzle the olive oil into a pan and place over a medium heat. Add the onions, cover with a lid and cook for 8 – 10 minutes until soft (stirring occasionally). Add the apple juice and raisins and cook (without the lid) over a medium heat for 10 minutes. Add the balsamic vinegar and continue to cook (with the lid off) for a further 10 minutes until most of the vinegar has evaporated and the mixture thickens. Turn off the heat and transfer to a little dish.

SERVE:

Great either warm or cold to accompany most dishes, but works particularly well with a lovely goats cheese salad — see page 81.

LEMON PESTO DRESSING

ROUGHLY
2 MINS

Ridiculously simple to make and yet so stupidly delicious and good for you. If you've never made fresh pesto before, once you've whizzed this up, you'll wonder why anyone ever buys the stuff in a jar!

GLUTEN-FREE

VEGETARIAN

CONTAINS NUTS

INGREDIENTS:

(Perfect for 2 generous servings)

Fresh Basil
30g or 1 handful
Parmesan or Parmigiano Reggiano Cheese*
35g or 1oz
Pine Nuts
30g or 1 small handful
Olive Oil
4 tablespoons
Lemon (the juice of)
1
Himalayan Rock Salt
1 pinch
Ground Black Pepper
1 generous pinch

PREPARE:

Remove the leaves from the basil and discard the stalks (unless you have a very good blender!). Roughly chop the cheese. Put all the ingredients in the larger blending container that accompanies a hand blender or you can use a *Retro Super Blend* or 'bullet' style blender.

BLEND:

Blitz for about 30 seconds.

*If vegan, use 4 tablespoons of nutritional yeast.

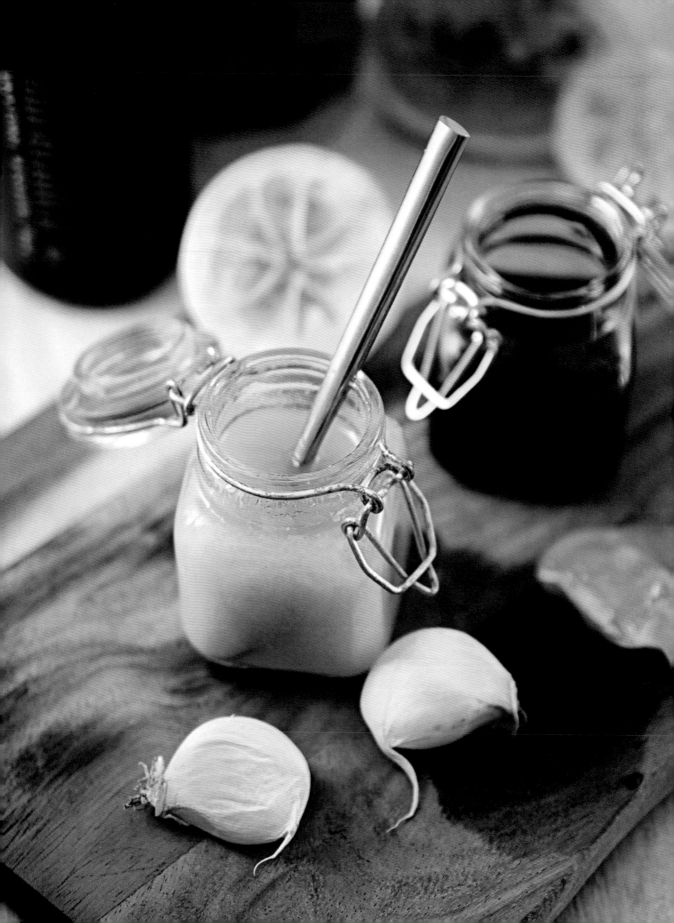

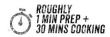
ORANGE & BALSAMIC REDUCTION

In my opinion, orange and balsamic vinegar were destined to be together and this dressing will help to lift any salad. It takes a little time to prepare, so I would make a double or triple batch and then store for another day.

GLUTEN-FREE

VEGAN

VEGETARIAN

INGREDIENTS:

Makes about 40ml/1.5fl oz, perfect to dress 2 salads

Oranges
2
Balsamic Vinegar
4 tablespoons

PREPARE:

Squeeze the juice of the oranges directly into a small saucepan.

REDUCE:

Add the vinegar to the pan and gently simmer (with the lid off) for 30 minutes, until the mixture has reduced and thickened a little.

TIP:

Wash the pan as soon as possible!

ROASTED GARLIC, LEMON & HONEY DRESSING

I was going to call it the 'anti-inflammatory' dressing, as garlic is one of the world's best natural anti-inflammatories. However, I thought the ingredients themselves sounded much more tantalizing! This dressing hits the mark nutritionally and gives any dish that often much needed bite.

GLUTEN-FREE

VEGAN

VEGETARIAN

INGREDIENTS:

Serves 2

Garlic
2 cloves (skin on)
Lemon (the juice of)
½
Olive Oil
3 tablespoons
Honey*
1 teaspoon

* If vegan please use an alternative sweetener.

PREPARE:

Preheat the oven to 180 °C (350 °F / gas mark 4).

ROAST:

Place the cloves of garlic onto a baking tray with the skin on and cook for 5 minutes.

MAKE:

Remove the garlic from the oven and carefully peel (it's hot!) and remove any hard ends. Place the garlic, lemon juice, oil and honey into the small mixing container of a hand blender, *Super Blend* or 'bullet' style blender.

BLITZ:

Blitz for 20 seconds.

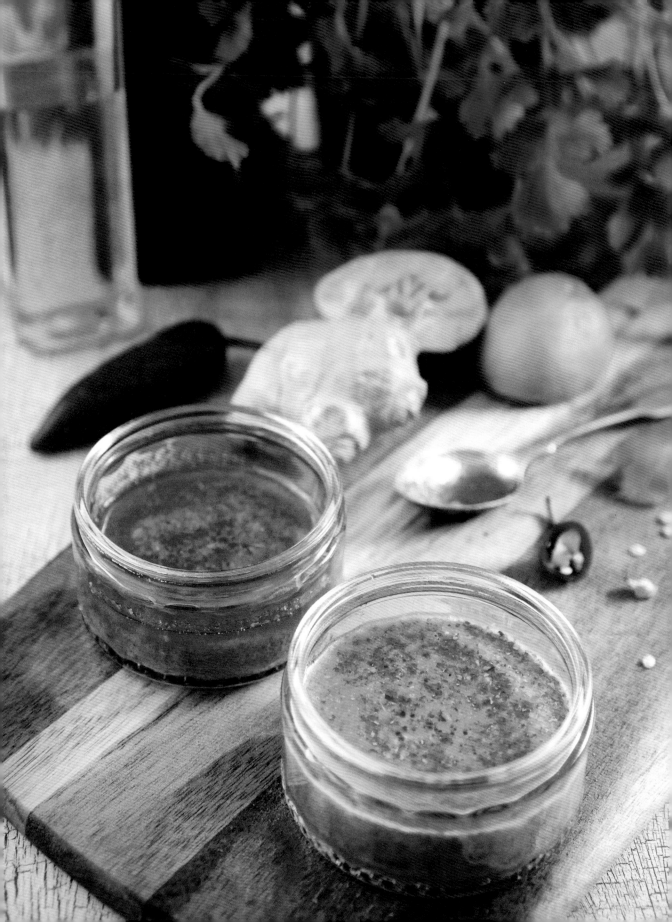

LIME, CHILLI & CORIANDER DRESSING

LOVE this dressing! It has a wonderful fire to it that is balanced beautifully by the zest of the lime and the fragrance of coriander.

GLUTEN-FREE

VEGAN

VEGETARIAN

INGREDIENTS:

Serves 2

Red Chilli
1 medium
Fresh Coriander
20g or 1 small handful
Apple Cider Vinegar
1 tablespoon
Olive Oil
3 tablespoons
Lime (the juice of)
½

PREPARE:

Remove the top from the chilli, slice in half lengthways, discard the seeds and place in the mixing container of a hand blender, 'bullet' or *Retro Super Blend*, along with all the other ingredients.

WHIZZ:

Blitz for 10 – 20 seconds.

GINGER, CHILLI & SESAME DRESSING

Quick and easy to make and helps to add a beautiful fiery edge to any salad. I also love this as a dipping sauce to accompany some warm, sweet potato wedges.

GLUTEN-FREE

VEGAN

VEGETARIAN

INGREDIENTS:

Serves 2

Chilli
1 medium
Fresh Ginger
20g or 2 cm x 2 cm
Sesame Oil
3 tablespoons
Apple Cider Vinegar
1 tablespoon

PREPARE:

Remove the top from the chilli, cut in half lengthways, discard the seeds and place in a 'bullet' style blender, *Retro Super Blend* or the small mixing container of a hand blender. Peel the ginger, chop into chunks and add to the mixing container along with the oil and vinegar.

BLEND:

Blitz for 30 — 60 seconds until all the ingredients are blended.

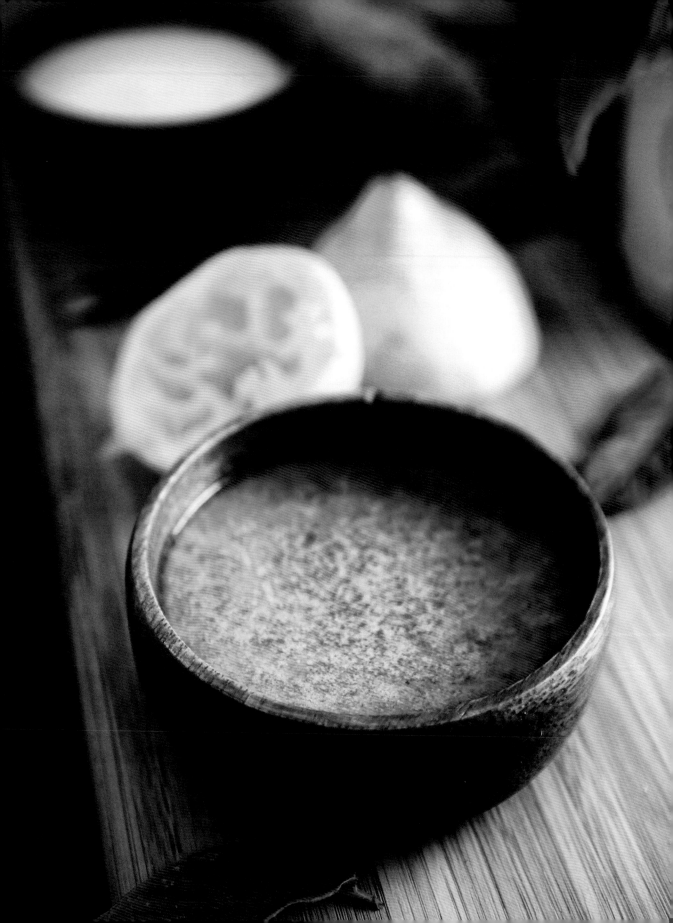

GINGER, HONEY & YOGURT SPLASH

A cool, sweet and slightly fiery, combination to help beautifully compliment many a dish.

GLUTEN-FREE

VEGETARIAN

INGREDIENTS:

Serves 2

Fresh Ginger
10g or 1 cm x 2 cm
Natural Yogurt
3 tablespoons
Honey
1 teaspoon

INSTRUCTIONS:

Peel the ginger, chop and place in the small mixing container of a hand blender, *Retro Super Blend* or 'bullet' style blender. Add the yogurt and honey.

MIX:

Blend for about 20 seconds.

TAHINI, LEMON & MINT DRESSING

Loaded with B vitamins, amino acids and fatty acids, this dressing is more than just a pretty face. It's thicker than your average dressing and goes nicely with most salads.

GLUTEN-FREE

VEGAN

VEGETARIAN

INGREDIENTS:

(serves 2)

Fresh Mint
20g or 1 small handful
Lemon (the juice of)
½
Tahini
2 tablespoons
Olive Oil
3 tablespoons

PREPARE:

Remove the leaves from the mint, discard the stems and place in the small container of a hand blender, *Retro Super Blend* or 'bullet' style blender. Add the lemon juice, tahini and olive oil.

WHIZZ:

Blend for about 20 seconds.

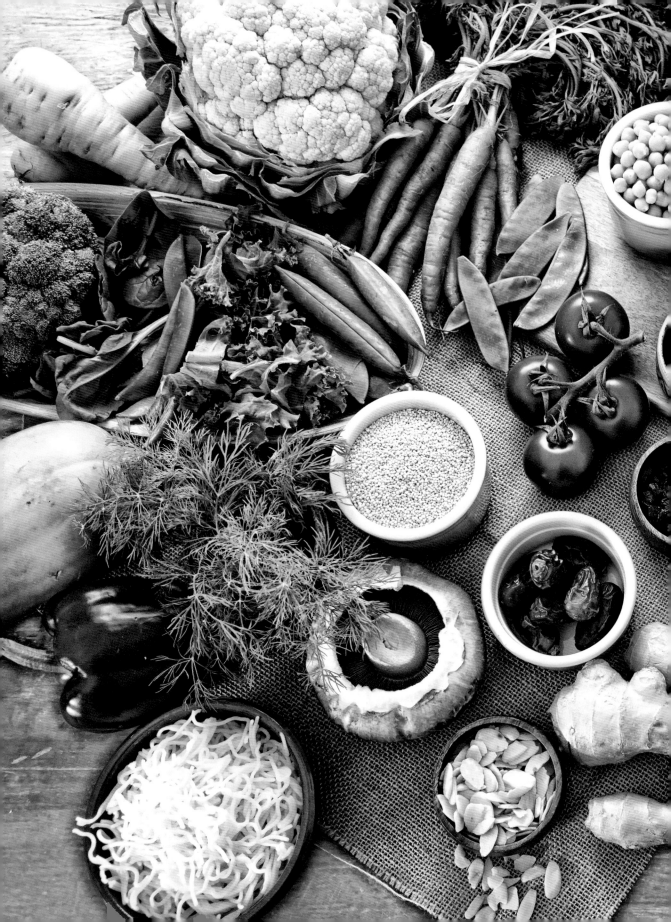

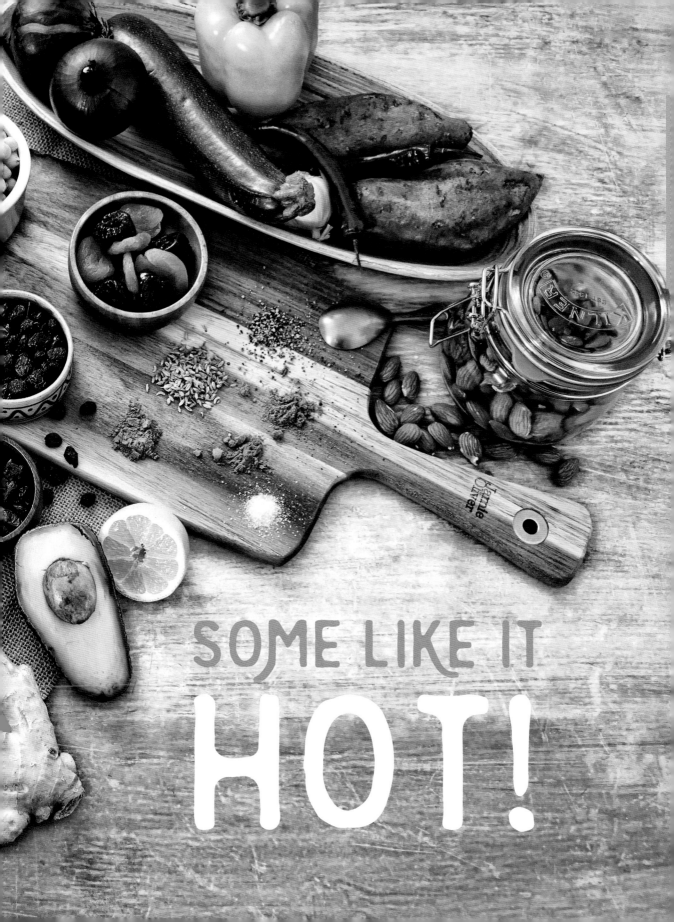

SOME LIKE IT
HOT!

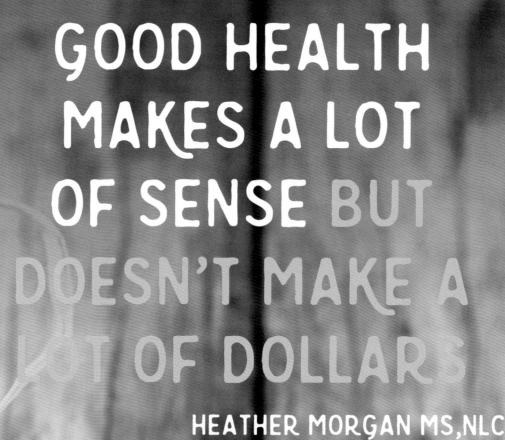

GOOD HEALTH MAKES A LOT OF SENSE BUT DOESN'T MAKE A LOT OF DOLLARS

HEATHER MORGAN MS,NLC

VEGAN
PUT YOUR HAND UP IF YOU'RE A VEGAN
(IF YOU'VE GOT THE STRENGTH THAT IS!)

There are two main misconceptions about being vegan and vegan food in general. One is that vegan food is bland and boring the other is that vegan food is lacking in nutrients, especially protein. However, we need to understand that the largest land animals on earth with the greatest muscle mass, tend to be vegan (think elephants, rhinos, bullocks, etc.) All of their protein is built from the amino acids found in their plant based diet and is more than sufficient to build and maintain their often huge muscle mass. Now clearly our constitutions are different to that of an elephant for example, but our protein, like theirs, is also built from amino acids. Meaning, like elephants, all of our protein requirements can be met through vegan food too. The good news is, unlike in the wild where vegan food is indeed pretty boring and monotonous; us humans have managed to conjure up some pretty wonderful vegan dishes bursting with flavor and overflowing with genuine nutrients. Once you make the recipes in this section I hope you'll agree that going vegan doesn't mean going bland or boring!

Here you'll find:

* BUTTERNUT SQUASH, CHILLI, LIME & COCONUT CURRY ON A BED OF CAULIFLOWER 'RICE' (page 125)
* VEGETABLE & CHICKPEA TAGINE SERVED WITH WARM FRUITY QUINOA (page 127)
* SWEET POTATO CAKES WITH ALMOND LEMON DRIZZLE (page 129)
* GRIDDLED AVOCADO, TOMATO & MUSHROOM WITH A SIDE OF STEAMED GREENS (page 133)

I was a vegan for over four years and I am sorry to say that a cheese sandwich broke me at an airport! However, the vast majority of my diet remains largely vegan and veggie based and why wouldn't it when you can make vegan dishes that taste this good!

Remember to snap a pic of whichever vegan dish you decide to make and share it on social media to spread the Super *fast* Food message and help to make a difference.

#superfastfood

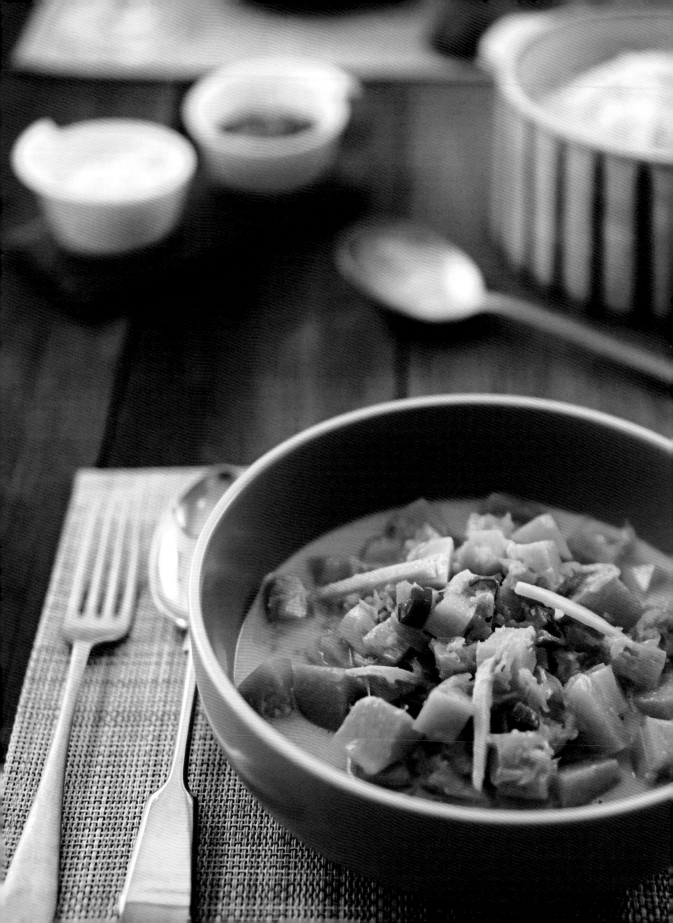

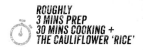

BUTTERNUT SQUASH, CHILLI, LIME & COCONUT CURRY ON A BED OF CAULIFLOWER 'RICE'

GLUTEN-FREE

VEGAN

VEGETARIAN

Cauliflower 'rice' is an alternative for anyone who, for whatever reason, wants something a little different to traditional rice. Cauliflower contains vitamins B1 (thiamine), B2 (riboflavin), B3 (niacin), B5 (pantothenic acid), B6 (pyridoxine) and B9 (folic acid), as well as omega-3 fatty acids and vitamin K. It serves as a good source of protein, phosphorus and potassium. All of which add up to a good reason to try it, plus it tastes pretty delicious too. This curry has a kick in all the right places without being too overpowering and is the perfect hot dish for a cold winter's night.

INGREDIENTS:

Serves 2

Butternut Squash
½ medium

Red Onion
½ medium

Red Chilli
1 medium

Garlic
2 cloves

Fresh Ginger
30g or 2 cm x 4 cm

Coconut Oil
1 tablespoon

Coconut Milk
400ml/14fl oz or 1 tin

Ground Turmeric
½ level teaspoon

Lime (the juice of)
1

Cauliflower 'Rice'*
Page 217

PREPARE:

Remove the ends from the butternut squash, peel and then chop into bite sized chunks about 1 cm x 1 cm (discarding the seeds). Remove the ends and skin from the red onion and then slice thinly. Remove the top from the chilli, cut in half and then cut into thin slices. Remove the ends and skin from the garlic and thinly slice. Peel the ginger and then cut into pieces the size of matchsticks.

COOK:

Put the coconut oil in a wok (or large frying pan) and place over a medium heat. Add the butternut squash and cook for 10 minutes, stirring occasionally, then add the onion, chilli, garlic and ginger and cook for a further 5 minutes. Next add the coconut milk, turmeric and lime juice to the pan. Reduce the heat and allow to simmer for a further 10 minutes.

MEANWHILE:

Make the cauliflower 'rice'* — page 217

SERVE:

Scoop a generous spoonful or two of the 'rice' and curry into your bowl.

*You can use regular rice if you prefer and simply cook this according to the packet instructions.

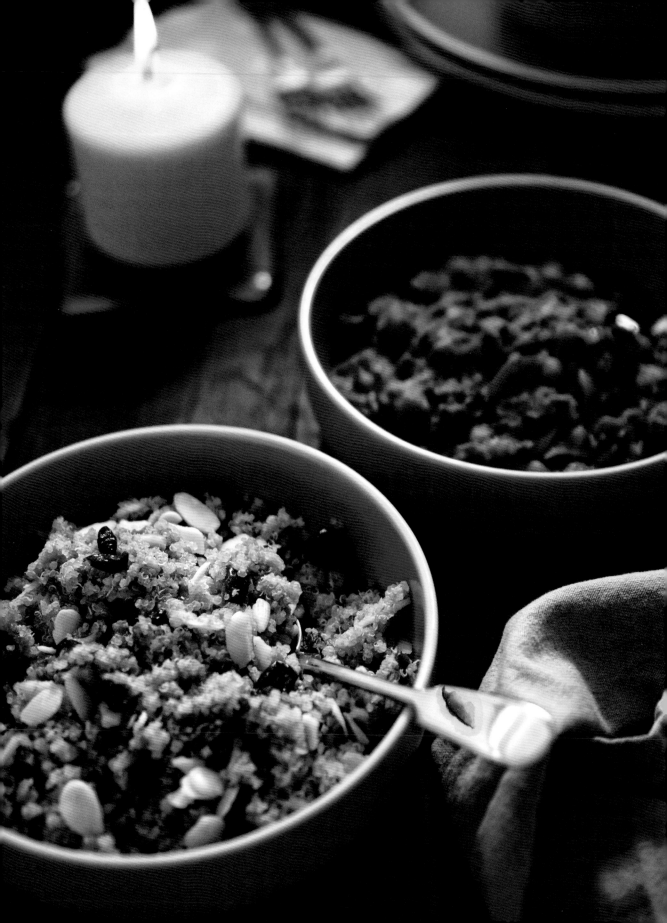

GLUTEN-FREE

VEGAN

VEGETARIAN

VEGETABLE & CHICKPEA TAGINE SERVED WITH WARM FRUITY QUINOA

Sweet, succulent, aromatic, warm, fruity and filling are all words which capture the true essence of this delightful Moroccan dish. Another superfood combination which provides comfort, without the calories. Ok, so this one takes a little longer to make than some of the other recipes (so you may want to sue me for the 'fast' bit in the main title of the book!) but good things really do come to those who wait, and once you taste it you won't mind, it's *that* good! It's also rich in protein, essential fats, vitamins, minerals, phytonutrients and antioxidants, all adding up to time well spent.

INGREDIENTS:

Serves 2

Red Onion
½ medium

Red Pepper
1 medium

Sweet Potato
1 medium

Chickpeas (tinned)
200g/7oz or ½ tin

Fresh Ginger
30g or 2 cm x 4 cm chunk

Prunes
60g/2oz

Warm Fruity Quinoa
Page 225

Olive Oil
1 tablespoon

Ground Cinnamon
1 teaspoon

Ground Turmeric
1 teaspoon

Boiling Water
400ml/14fl oz

Honey*
1 tablespoon

PREPARE:

Remove the ends and skin from the onion and cut into small chunks. Cut the red pepper in half, remove the core and cut into pieces roughly the same size as the onion. Peel the sweet potato and chop into cubes roughly 1 cm x 1 cm. Drain and rinse the chickpeas (if using raw chickpeas, soak and cook as per the packet instructions). Peel the ginger and grate using a fine grater. Remove the stones from the prunes and cut into quarters.

Make the Warm Fruity Quinoa — page 225

COOK:

Heat the olive oil in a pan over a medium heat and add the onion, pepper, sweet potato, grated ginger, cinnamon and turmeric. Cook for 5 minutes, stirring constantly and then add the water and chickpeas, reduce the heat and simmer for 30 minutes (with the lid off). Finally add the prunes and honey and allow to simmer for a further 2 minutes. Remove from the heat and using a hand stick blender, pulse for just 10 seconds, so that some of the tagine gets blended while the rest remains intact.

SERVE:

Heap the quinoa onto the plate and add a generous spoonful of tagine.

*If vegan please use an alternative sweetener.

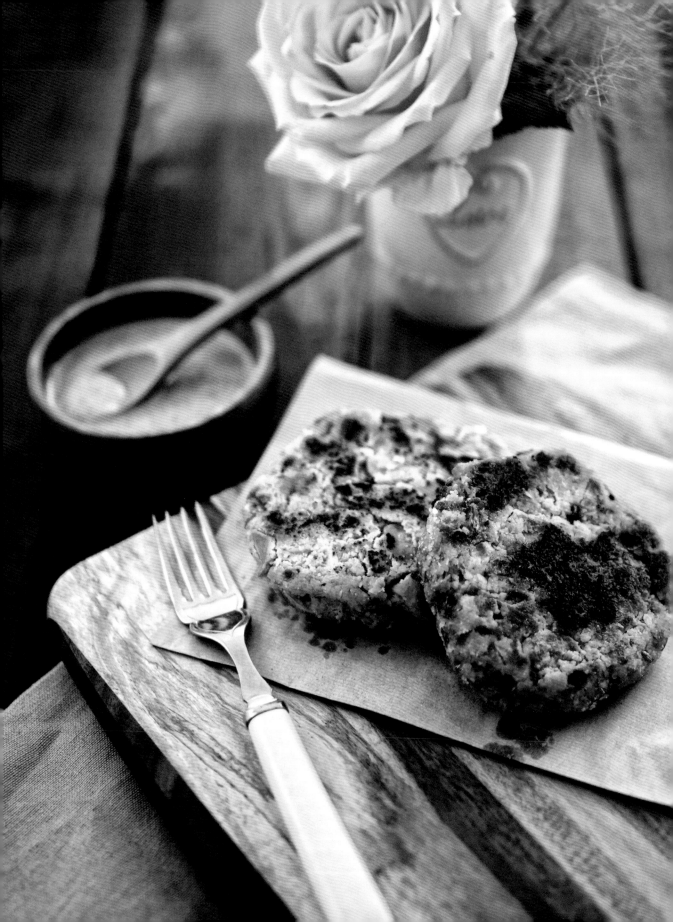

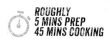
SWEET POTATO CAKES WITH AN ALMOND LEMON DRIZZLE

GLUTEN-FREE

VEGAN

VEGETARIAN

CONTAINS NUTS

If you have recently ventured down the vegan path and used to love fishcakes, then this vegan friendly recipe is the perfect alternative. They work well as a dish in themselves, or why not add a cheeky side order of sweet potato wedges to raise the game. This simple recipe will feed you from the inside out with its generous quantities of vitamins A, B6, C, E and minerals including calcium, iron and magnesium.

POTATO CAKE INGREDIENTS:

Serves 2

Sweet Potatoes
2 medium

Carrot
1 medium

Red Onion
½ medium

Garlic
2 cloves

Almonds
100g or 2 handfuls

Fennel Seeds
1 tablespoon

Olive Oil
1 tablespoon

Himalayan Rock Salt
1 pinch

Ground Black Pepper
1 generous pinch

DRIZZLE INGREDIENTS:

Lemon (the juice of)
¼

Water
1 tablespoon

Almond Butter
2 teaspoons

POTATO CAKE PREP:

Preheat the oven to 180 °C (350 °F/gas mark 4).

Peel the sweet potatoes and carrot and remove the hard ends. Remove the ends and skin from the onion. Peel the garlic. Chop the sweet potatoes, carrot and onion into small chunks.

Using either a food processor or a compact style blender, blitz the almonds and fennel seeds for 10 – 20 seconds until they turn into 'flour'.

COOK:

Put the sweet potato, carrot, onion and garlic onto a baking tray, drizzle with the olive oil, stir so all the veg are coated and place in the oven for 30 minutes, stirring part way through.

MEANWHILE MAKE THE DRIZZLE:

Put the lemon juice into an old jar; add the water and almond butter and shake well to combine.

CREATE THE POTATO CAKES:

Put the cooked vegetables, almond 'flour', salt and pepper into a pan (but keep the baking tray out and do not turn the oven off) and mash using a potato masher. Divide the mixture and shape into 4 'burgers', place on the baking tray and pop back in the oven.

COOK:

Cook for 15 minutes.

SERVE:

Drizzle the dressing over the potato cakes.

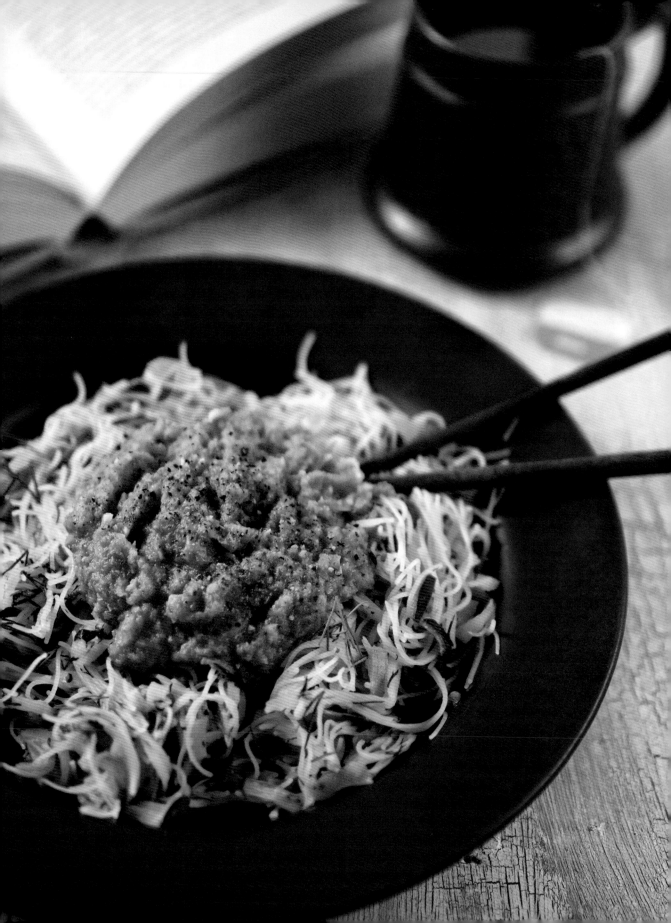

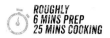
FRESH VEGGIE NOODLES WITH A ROASTED PEPPER SAUCE

This dish is extremely easy to make and stupidly good for you. I LOVE rice noodles and find, unlike many carbs, they don't ever bloat. This is such a light dish, yet surprisingly satisfying and the combination of flavours work beautifully. As you'd expect, the superfood element has been addressed with garlic, onion, pepper, carrot, courgette and parsnip all making a showing.

GLUTEN-FREE

VEGAN

VEGETARIAN

INGREDIENTS FOR THE VEGGIE NOODLES:

Serves 2

Courgette
1 medium

Carrot
1 medium

Parsnip
1 medium

Fresh Dill
10g or 1 small handful

Boiling Water
1 litre/35fl oz

Rice Noodles (wide flat ones if possible)
300g/11oz

Himalayan Rock Salt
1 pinch

Ground Pepper
1 generous pinch

INGREDIENTS FOR THE ROASTED PEPPER SAUCE:

Red Pepper
2 medium

Yellow Pepper
2 medium

Red Onion
1 medium

Garlic
2 cloves

Olive Oil
1 tablespoon

Apple Cider Vinegar
1 tablespoon

PREPARE THE NOODLES:

Preheat the oven to 180 °C (350 °F/gas mark 4).

If you have a spiralizer, then spiralize the courgette, carrot and parsnip and place in a saucepan. Alternatively you can finely cut these vegetables into very thin strips. Finely chop the dill, removing any hard stalks.

PREPARE THE SAUCE:

Cut the peppers into quarters and remove the cores. Remove the ends and skin from the onion and garlic. Cut the onion into quarters and place the peppers, onion and garlic onto a baking tray. Drizzle with the olive oil.

ROAST:

Place the baking tray in the oven and roast for 25 minutes.

MAKE THE NOODLES:

5 minutes before the roasted vegetables are cooked, pour the boiling water over the courgette, carrot and parsnip, cover with a lid and cook over a medium heat for 4 minutes, then remove from the heat, add the rice noodles, replace the lid and leave for 1 minute. Next strain away the water, return to the pan, add the dill, salt and pepper, stir gently and replace the lid.

MAKE THE SAUCE:

Place the roasted vegetables into either a food processor or the blender container of a stick blender. Add the apple cider vinegar and blend for 60 seconds until everything turns into a sauce.

SERVE:

Spoon the noodle dish into a bowl, pour over the sauce and enjoy.

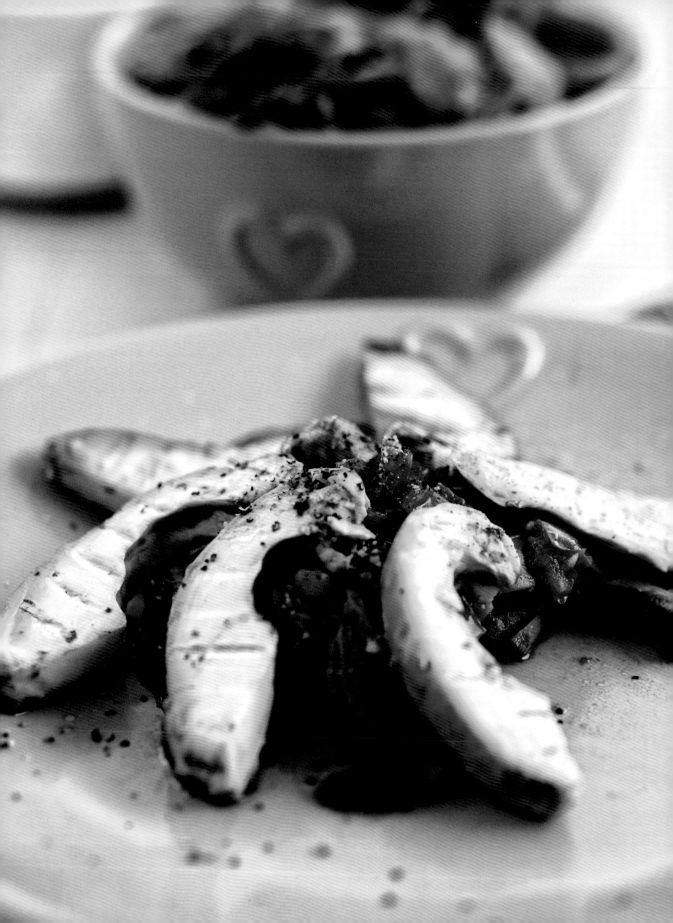

GRIDDLED AVOCADO, TOMATO & MUSHROOM WITH A SIDE OF STEAMED GREENS

GLUTEN-FREE

VEGAN

VEGETARIAN

My lovely Katie has assured me that most people will love this recipe and that if I liked mushrooms I would too. Firstly, thank you Katie for once again adding your natural cooking prowess to this recipe book and secondly, I'll just have to take your word for it! I hate mushrooms, like really hate them and therefore, I will never personally try this dish as intended. However, I have tried it without the mushrooms and it tastes pretty damn good. If you are a mushroom lover, I've got it on very good authority, you'll love this combo. Quick and easy to make and 'off the scale' good for you, due to the superfood king avocado making a showing!

INGREDIENTS:

Serves 2

Steamed Greens with Chilli & Fennel
Page 209
Avocados (ripe)
2 medium
Tomatoes
3 medium
Portobello or Large Mushrooms
2
Sesame Oil
2 tablespoons
Ground Black Pepper
1 generous pinch
Himalayan Salt
1 pinch

PREPARE:

Make the Steamed Greens — page 209

Cut the avocados in half, discard the stone, remove the flesh, and cut into thick slices about 1 cm wide. Dice the tomatoes. Wash and dry the mushrooms and cut into slices about 1 cm thick. Put the mushrooms on a plate, drizzle with the oil and turn to ensure both sides are coated.

GRIDDLE:

Warm a griddle pan till it is lovely and hot, then add the mushrooms and cook for 3 minutes, before turning and adding the avocados and tomatoes to the griddle. Cook the avocados for 1 minute each side. Stir the tomatoes.

SERVE:

Place the mushrooms, followed by the tomatoes and finish with the avocados in a little stack on a plate, sprinkle over the black pepper and salt and accompany with the steamed greens.

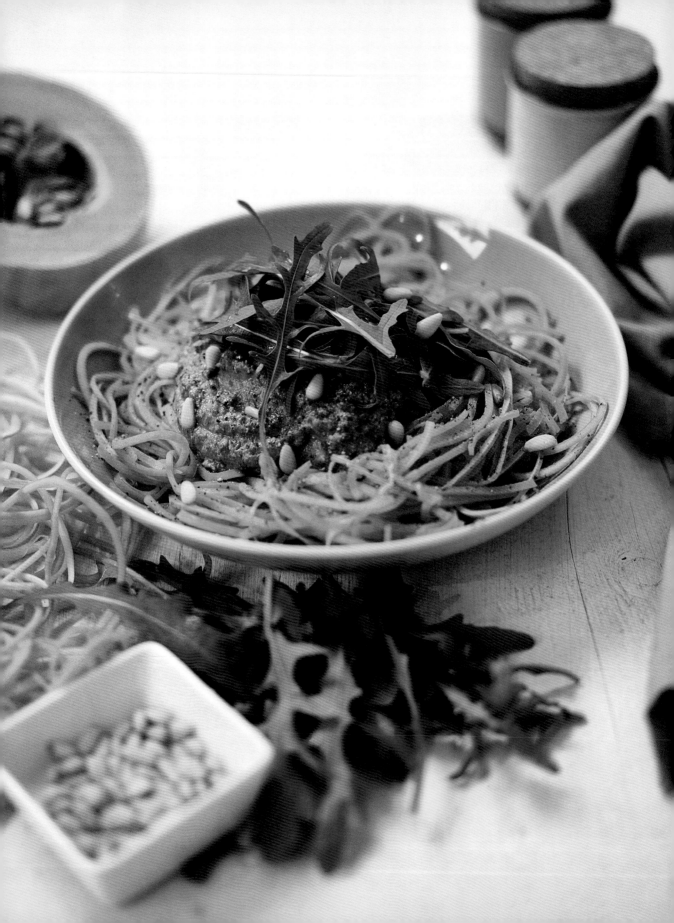

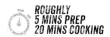

BUTTERNUT SQUASH AL DENTE 'PASTA' WITH ROASTED RED PEPPER PESTO

This is a great alternative for anyone who wishes to steer clear of regular pasta for whatever reason. Clearly it's not pasta, it's butternut squash which has been spiralized to look like pasta, but I'm sure the non pedantic amongst you won't mind me calling it pasta. The hero of this dish however, is not the butternut squash 'pasta', but rather the roasted red pepper pesto. As homemade pasta sauces go, this really is something special. All of the ingredients are natural and super in their own right, but combine them together and you get a plethora of nature's finest flavours, all working beautifully together to feed every cell in the body. This dish is bursting with colour and won't make you feel bloated, which is often the case with regular wheat pasta.

GLUTEN-FREE

VEGAN

VEGETARIAN

CONTAINS NUTS

INGREDIENTS:

Serves 2

Butternut Squash
1 small
Red Peppers
2
Olive Oil
5 tablespoons
Garlic Cloves (with skin on)
2
Pine Nuts
50g / 2 oz
Water
200ml / 7 fl oz
Himalayan Rock Salt
1 pinch
Ground Black Pepper
1 pinch
Sun-dried Tomatoes
100g / 3.5 oz
Rocket Leaves
30g / 1 oz

PREPARE:

Preheat the oven to 180 °C (350 °F / gas mark 4)

Peel the butternut squash and spiralize. Remove the core and seeds from the peppers and chop into quarters.

COOK:

Put 1 tablespoon of olive oil in a baking tray, add the red peppers and pop in the oven for 15 minutes. Then turn the peppers, add the garlic, pine nuts and cook for a further 5 minutes.

MEANWHILE:

Put 1 tablespoon of olive oil into a large pan over a medium heat, add the butternut squash and cook for 3 minutes stirring constantly. Then add the water, salt, pepper and continue cooking for a further 5 minutes or until the water has evaporated. Remove from the heat, cover with a lid and set to one side.

CREATE THE PESTO:

Remove the baking tray from the oven. Carefully peel the garlic (watch out, it's hot!) and place in the container of a hand blender or *Retro Super Blend / Bullet*. Add the peppers, sundried tomatoes, half the pine nuts, the remaining olive oil and pulse until all the ingredients are combined.

SERVE:

Scoop the butternut squash onto a plate, add the pesto, a handful of rocket and finish with a sprinkling of toasted pine nuts.

NOTHING WILL BENEFIT
HUMAN HEALTH AND
INCREASE THE CHANCES OF
SURVIVAL OF LIFE ON EARTH
AS MUCH AS THE EVOLUTION
TO A VEGETARIAN DIET.

ALBERT EINSTEIN

VEGETARIAN
PEOPLE EAT MEAT THINKING THEY WILL BECOME AS STRONG AS AN OX, FORGETTING THAT THE OX EATS GRASS!

More and more people are starting to turn to the veggie side of life as evidence suggests that going veggie is better for your health. However, many are fearful of doing so as they feel their diet will become far less fulfilling and pretty dull. One of my friends, who seemingly followed this belief system, once put it like this, 'I would go veggie but I'd rather have a shorter yet happier life than one where I only eat green leaves every day!' I see where he is coming from, but vegetarian dining is now so far removed from the 'rabbit food' era, as good vegetarian dishes go way beyond the 'green leaf' and are often even much more flavorsome and fulfilling than their meaty competition.

If you are a meat eater reading this, I am hoping the recipes in this section help you to see that **a meal without meat is far from a sacrifice** and will **introduce you to a whole new world of exciting textures and fuller flavors**. If you are already a vegetarian, then I'm hoping you'll find some new inspiration within the next pages that will hit all of your veggie buttons and help to mix things up a bit! In this section you'll find one of my favorite recipes of the whole book — the **Grilled Halloumi Vegetable Stack with a Drizzle of Lemon Pesto** (page 139) — this, in my opinion, is to die for!

You'll also find:

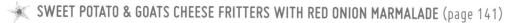

* **SWEET POTATO & GOATS CHEESE FRITTERS WITH RED ONION MARMALADE** (page 141)
* **PUREED PEA & MINT RISOTTO WITH WILD ROCKET & BALSAMIC** (page 143)
* **'THYME' FOR VEGGIE BAKE WITH MELTED MOZZARELLA** (page 145)
* **SUPER CHARGED EGG FRIED RICE** (page 147)

All of these veggie friendly recipes have been designed to be incredibly satisfying, bursting with flavor as well as quick and easy to make. As with all the recipes in the book it's a case of **No Chef Required**.

Remember to snap a pic of whichever veggie dish takes your fancy and share it on social media to spread the **Super *fast* Food** message and help to make a difference.

#superfastfood

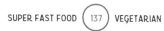

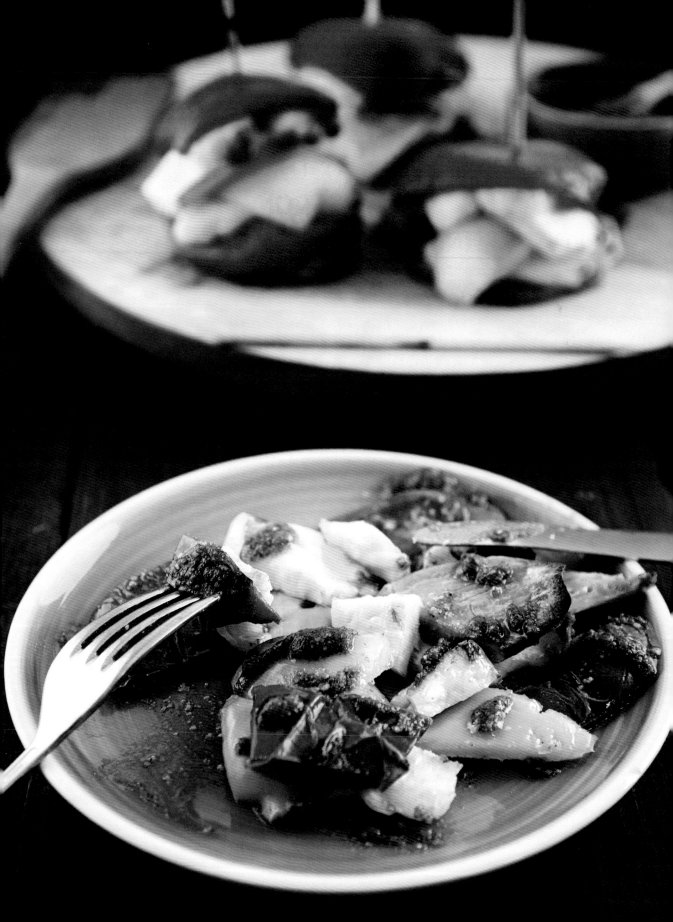

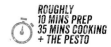

GRILLED HALLOUMI VEGETABLE STACK WITH A DRIZZLE OF LEMON PESTO

GLUTEN-FREE

VEGETARIAN

CONTAINS NUTS

YOU HAVE TO MAKE THIS ONE! Yes, I am aware I am shouting, but there are certain recipes in the book I don't want you to miss out on and this 'are you kidding me?!' dish is one of them. It hits every taste bud button you would ever want and the key is make sure every part of the 'stack' is on your fork before it enters your mouth. I'll be frank here, I am trying to write this description when all I really want to do is make it and eat it! I know it's always good to under promise and over deliver, but sod that — this baby is SO, SO, SO GOOD! Yes, it's good for you, but taste is the overriding winner here — ENJOY!

INGREDIENTS:

Serves 2

Courgette/Zucchini
½ medium

Red Pepper
1 small

Yellow Pepper
1 small

Beef Tomato
1

Sweet Potato
1 small

Halloumi
250g/9oz

Olive Oil
2 tablespoons

Wooden Skewers
4

Lemon Pesto Dressing
Page 113

PREPARE:

Preheat the oven to 180 °C (350 °F/gas mark 4).

Remove the ends from the courgette and peel. Cut the courgette lengthways into 4 slices. Cut the peppers into quarters and remove the seeds. Remove the ends from the beef tomato and cut into 4 slices. Peel the sweet potato and cut lengthways into 4 slices. Cut the halloumi into 8 slices.

COOK:

Drizzle ½ tablespoon of olive oil on a baking tray (making sure the tray is covered). Place the sweet potato on the tray with as much room around each piece as possible, then drizzle another ½ tablespoon of olive oil over the slices. Place in the oven for 10 minutes.

MEANWHILE...

Make 4 kebabs by adding the ingredients in the following order to each skewers – red pepper; halloumi; courgette; yellow pepper; halloumi and finish with the tomato. Then remove the baking tray from the oven and turn the potatoes over. Next place a loaded kebab skewer into each potato to form a stack with the red pepper on the top. Drizzle the remaining olive oil over the stacks. Return to the oven and cook for 25 minutes.

MEANWHILE...

Make the Lemon Pesto Dressing page 113.

SERVE:

Place 2 x stacks on each plate and drizzle over the Lemon Pesto Dressing.

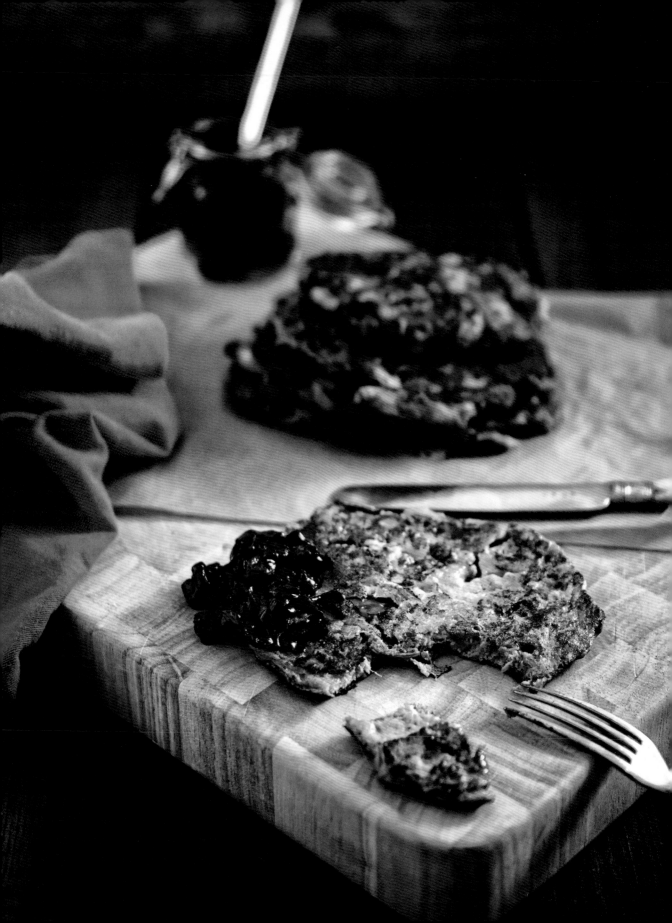

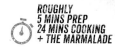

SWEET POTATO & GOATS CHEESE FRITTERS WITH RED ONION MARMALADE

GLUTEN-FREE

VEGETARIAN

These are SO nice! I really like sweet potato and I'm a big fan of goats cheese, but I'm disproportionately in love with how these already delicious ingredients are lifted by the stupidly good homemade Red Onion Marmalade. The fritters are perfect on their own, or with a nice side salad. Great as a main or a starter (adjust the ingredients accordingly) and surprisingly satisfying. They also pack one hell of a nutritional punch and are extremely easy to make. Hope you love as much as I!

INGREDIENTS:

Serves 2

Red Onion Marmalade
Page 113
Sweet Potatoes
2 medium
Red Onion
1 small
Garlic
2 cloves
Olive Oil
1 tablespoon
Goats Cheese (medium firmness)
100g/3.5oz
Eggs (free range & organic)
3 medium
Ground Cumin
2 teaspoons
Himalayan Rock Salt
1 pinch
Ground Black Pepper
1 generous pinch
Coconut Oil
1 teaspoon

PREPARE:

Preheat the oven to 180 °C (350 °C/gas mark 4).

Prepare the Red Onion Marmalade — page 113

Peel the sweet potatoes and chop into smallish chunks. Remove the ends and skin from the onion and dice. Peel the garlic. Place the potato, onions and garlic onto a baking tray, drizzle with the oil and toss so all the ingredients are coated. Cut the goats cheese into cubes. Whisk the eggs.

COOK:

Place the baking tray in the oven for 20 minutes, mixing part way through, then remove from the oven and place the ingredients in a saucepan.

COMBINE:

Add the cumin, salt and pepper to the pan and mash using a potato masher. When the mixture is all combined, add the eggs and mix. Then gently fold in the goats cheese, so it stays in chunks where possible.

COOK:

Put half the coconut oil in a frying pan over a medium to high heat, place a spoonful of the mixture in the pan and shape into a roundish fritters using the back of a spoon. Continue with the rest of the mixture until the pan is full (this will probably be just 2 or 3 fritters). Cook for 2 minutes one side, then turn and cook for 1 – 2 minutes on the other side until golden. Repeat with the rest of the coconut oil and mixture so you end up with 4 – 6 fritters.

SERVE:

Enjoy hot or cold with a generous spoonful of the red onion marmalade.

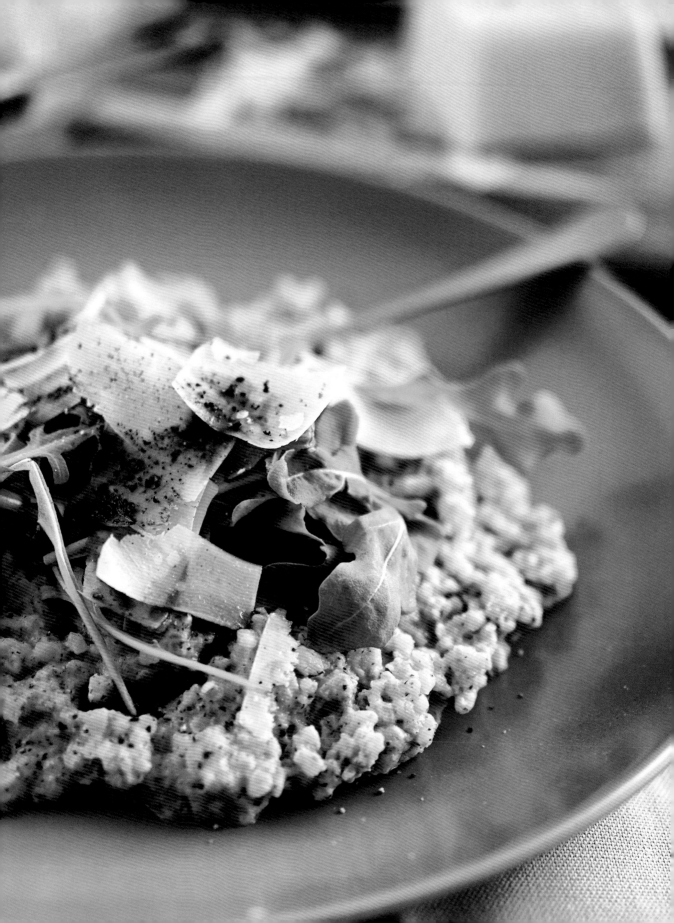

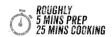
PUREED PEA & MINT RISOTTO WITH WILD ROCKET & BALSAMIC

GLUTEN-FREE

VEGETARIAN

If I was ever on a desert island and was only allowed one meal, this would be it. I don't like this recipe, I LOVE it a disproportionate amount (you know the 'get a room' type love it). This is a 'must make' recipe as it's easy, nutritious and delicious. Chlorophyll rich rocket adds a peppery punch and nudges up the nutrition in the form of powerful phytonutrients, vitamins A, C, K, folate and calcium. Seriously, whoever said being healthy meant eating tasteless food needed to have tried this!

INGREDIENTS:

Serves 2

Red Onion
½ medium
Garlic
2 cloves
Stock Cube
1
Boiling Water
600ml/21fl oz
Parmesan or Parmigiano Reggiano Cheese
75g/3oz
Olive Oil
1 tablespoon
Risotto Rice
200g/7oz
Himalayan Rock Salt
2 pinches
Ground Black Pepper
2 generous pinches
Peas
100g/3.5oz (fresh or frozen)
Boiling Water
200ml/7floz (for the peas)
Fresh Mint
30g or 1 large handful
Crème Fraîche
50ml/2fl oz
Wild Rocket
40g or 1 large handful
Balsamic Vinegar
½ tablespoon

PREPARE:

Remove the ends and skin from the onion and garlic and dice into very small pieces. Add the stock cube to the boiling water and stir. Using a vegetable peeler, thinly slice the cheese.

COOK:

Place the olive oil in a large pan and warm over a medium heat. Add the onion and garlic and cook for 5 minutes stirring frequently. Add the rice and cook for 2 minutes, stirring constantly. Add 200ml/7fl oz of the stock, 1 x pinch of salt and 1 x pinch of pepper, then reduce the heat and allow most of the water to absorb, stirring frequently. Keep adding 200ml/7fl oz of water at a time until it is all absorbed and the rice is cooked (you may need to add a little more water, if the rice is not completely cooked at this stage). When cooked, add half the cheese, stir well and remove from the heat.

MEANWHILE...

Place the peas in a small pan, cover with the boiling water (200ml/7fl oz) and boil for 5 minutes.

BLEND:

Drain the cooked peas, place in the mixing container of a hand blender or *Retro Super Blend* along with the mint and crème fraîche and blend for 30 seconds. Then add the pea puree and the remaining salt and pepper to the risotto and stir well.

SERVE:

Pile the risotto into a shallow bowl or plate, top with the rocket, the remaining cheese shavings and drizzle with the balsamic vinegar.

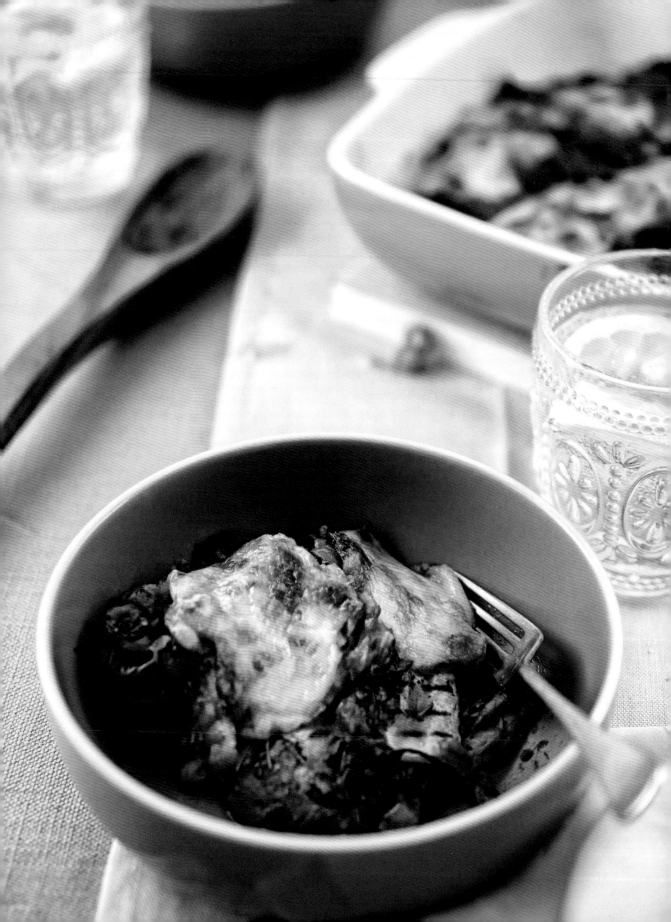

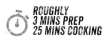

'THYME' FOR VEGGIE BAKE WITH MELTED MOZZARELLA

This is the perfect recipe for when you need a little warm comfort on a cold winter's eve but without the stodge. Despite the plethora of ingredients, it's incredibly easy to make and the whole dish takes less than 30 minutes. Some of the bad boys of the superfood world make a showing, such as garlic, tomato, spinach, thyme and red pepper, all combining to make it an extremely healthy dish. Remember, like all the recipes in this book, this makes enough for two. If you're making for one, be sure to halve the ingredients because trust me, this isn't one of those dishes where you'll be able to leave some for later!

INGREDIENTS:

Serves 2

Aubergine
1 small
Courgette
1 small
Leek
½ medium
Red Pepper
½ medium
Garlic
2 cloves
Tomatoes
4 x medium
Mozzarella
240g/8.5oz
Fresh Thyme
10g or 1 small handful
Olive Oil
1 tablespoon
Spinach
60g or 1 large handful
Himalayan Rock Salt
1 generous pinch
Ground Black Pepper
1 generous pinch

PREP:

Preheat the oven to 200 °C (400 °F/gas mark 6).

Remove the hard ends from the aubergine, courgette and leek. Remove the core and seeds from the red pepper. Peel the garlic. Cut the aubergine, courgette, leek, red pepper and garlic into smallish slices. Dice the tomato. Slice the mozzarella. Chop the thyme.

COOK:

Place a frying pan over a medium to high heat, add the olive oil, aubergine, courgette, leek, red pepper, garlic, tomatoes, thyme, spinach, salt and pepper and cook for 10 minutes, stirring frequently. Then transfer all the ingredients to an ovenproof dish, top with the mozzarella and cook for 15 minutes or until the mozzarella has browned.

SERVE:

Scoop onto a lovely plate or eat straight out of the baking dish!

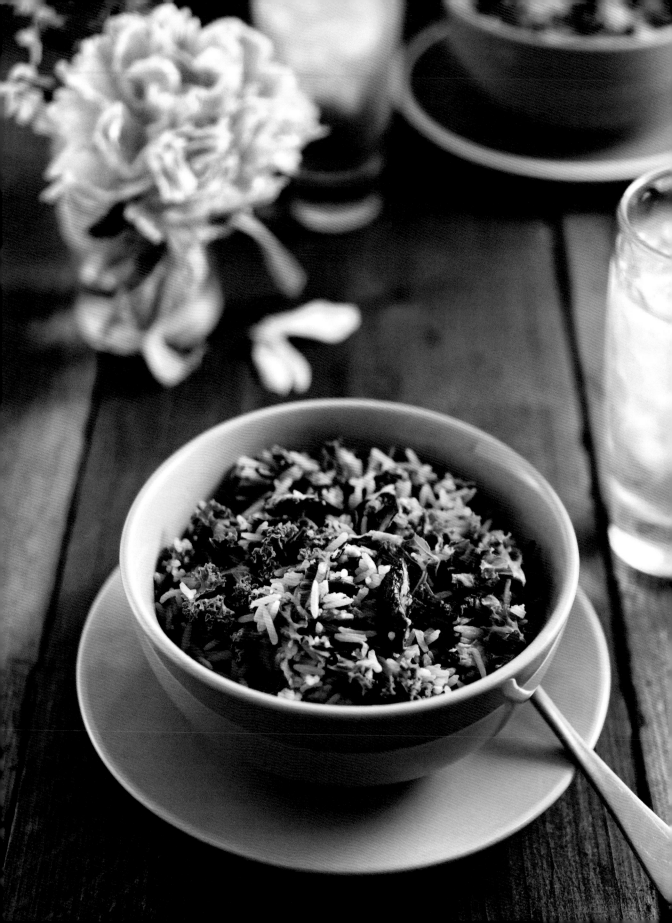

SUPER-CHARGED EGG FRIED RICE

This takes the classic egg fried rice to a whole new level, a Super *fast* Food level in fact! I love rice and it's a shame that quinoa has almost made this eastern staple a little unfashionable. It's loaded with essential nutrients, is a great source of fiber and good wild rice is easily worthy of superfood status on its own. However, add some kale, mushrooms, spring onions and pumpkin seeds and you've just raised the nutritional game a notch or two. I love this light and flavorsome version, but for me personally, the mushrooms take a back seat, as I'm just not a mushroom kind of guy. However, they're a great addition and this book is about creating beautiful superfood dishes for all...not just me.

GLUTEN-FREE

VEGETARIAN

INGREDIENTS:

Serves 2

Kale
50g or 1 handful

Mushrooms
4 medium

Spring Onions
4 sprigs

Eggs (free-range & organic obviously!)
4 medium

Mixed Wild Rice*
150g/5oz

Boiling Water
450ml/16fl oz

Sesame Oil
1 tablespoon

Soy Sauce**
1 tablespoon

Pumpkin Seeds
40g or 1 large handful

Ground Black Pepper
2 generous pinches

PREPARE:

Chop the kale into small pieces, discarding any hard stems. Wash the mushrooms and slice. Remove the ends and outer layer from the spring onion and cut into slices about 1 cm thick. Whisk the eggs. Rinse the rice, place in a pan and add the boiling water.

BOIL:

Place the rice on the hob and bring to the boil, then cover with a lid, reduce the heat and allow to simmer for 20 – 25 minutes until all the water has been absorbed. Keep checking the rice and add a little more water if the water is all absorbed and the rice is still not cooked. Once cooked, remove from heat, drain any excess water, place back in the pan and cover with a lid.

COOK:

Put the sesame oil in a wok or frying pan and heat over a medium to high heat. Add the kale, mushrooms and spring onions and cook for 5 minutes, stirring frequently. Add the eggs and allow to cook for 1 minute stirring constantly so that the eggs envelope all the ingredients and turn into scrambled eggs (and not an omelette!) Remove from the heat.

COMBINE:

Add the rice, soy sauce, pumpkin seeds and pepper to the frying pan and combine.

SERVE:

Place in a bowl and eat on your lap whilst sat in your favourite armchair.

* This will usually come in a bag with either basmati or wholegrain rice, it really doesn't matter which you use.

** If hyper sensitive to gluten use tamari or Braggs Liquid Aminos.

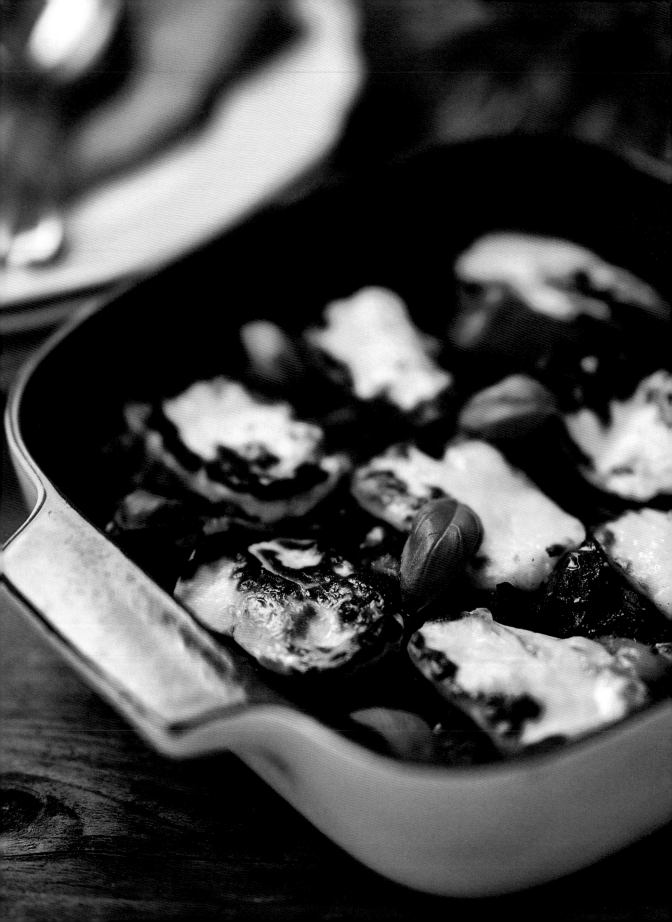

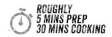
TOMATO, PEPPER & ROASTED NEW POTATOES WITH A GOLDEN BROWN HALLOUMI CROWN

GLUTEN-FREE

VEGETARIAN

If you haven't realised by now, I LOVE halloumi, which is why it gets top billing in this recipe. You can make this anytime of the year, but it really comes into its own on a cold winter's night in front of an open fire. It gives you that perfect warming, satisfying feeling without leaving you feeling bloated. It's also an effortless dinner party dish. Double up, or triple up on the ingredients and you can cook for many and even participate in the party yourself! The roasted vegetables are good but it's the final touch of grilled halloumi that really transforms this beautiful dish.

INGREDIENTS:

Serves 2

Olive Oil
2 tablespoons
New Potatoes
350g/12 oz
Himalayan Rock Salt
2 generous pinches
Ground Black Pepper
2 generous pinches
Orange Pepper
½
Yellow Pepper
½
Garlic
2 large cloves
Shallots
4 small
Tomatoes
(preferably red and orange
and yellow) 600g /21oz
Halloumi
250g/9 oz
Basil leaves
15g or 1 handful
Balsamic Vinegar
3 tablespoons

PREPARE:

Preheat the oven to 180 °C (350 °F / gas mark 4)

Place 1 tablespoon of olive oil into an ovenproof dish and pop in the oven to warm.

Cut the new potatoes into pieces (roughly 2–3 cm in size), then place in the warmed dish with 1 pinch of salt and pepper. Shake the dish to coat the potatoes in the oil and pop in the oven for 25 minutes, or until the potatoes are cooked. Remove the core from the peppers. Peel the garlic and shallots. Roughly chop the tomatoes, garlic, shallots and peppers. Slice the halloumi.

COOK:

Place the remaining olive oil in a frying pan and warm over a medium to high heat. Add the garlic, shallots and peppers and cook for a few minutes until they begin to brown. Then add the tomatoes, basil, balsamic vinegar and the remaining salt and pepper. Allow to cook for a further 10 minutes (stirring occasionally), or until the vegetables are cooked and the sauce has thickened.

Remove the potatoes from the oven and very gently smash some of the potatoes with a potato masher. Pour the tomato and pepper mix over the potatoes, top with the halloumi and pop under a hot grill for 5 minutes until the halloumi turns golden brown.

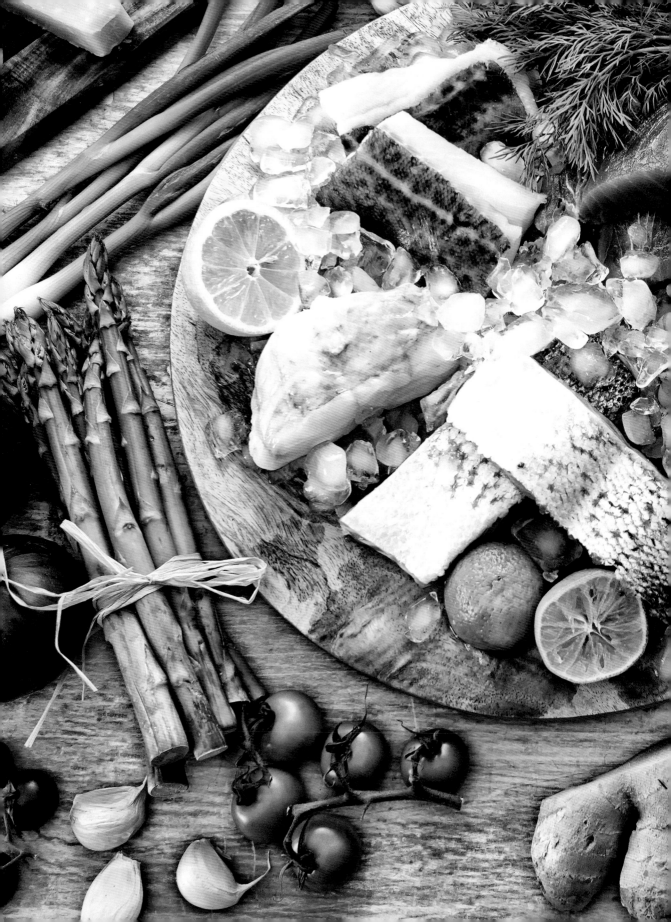

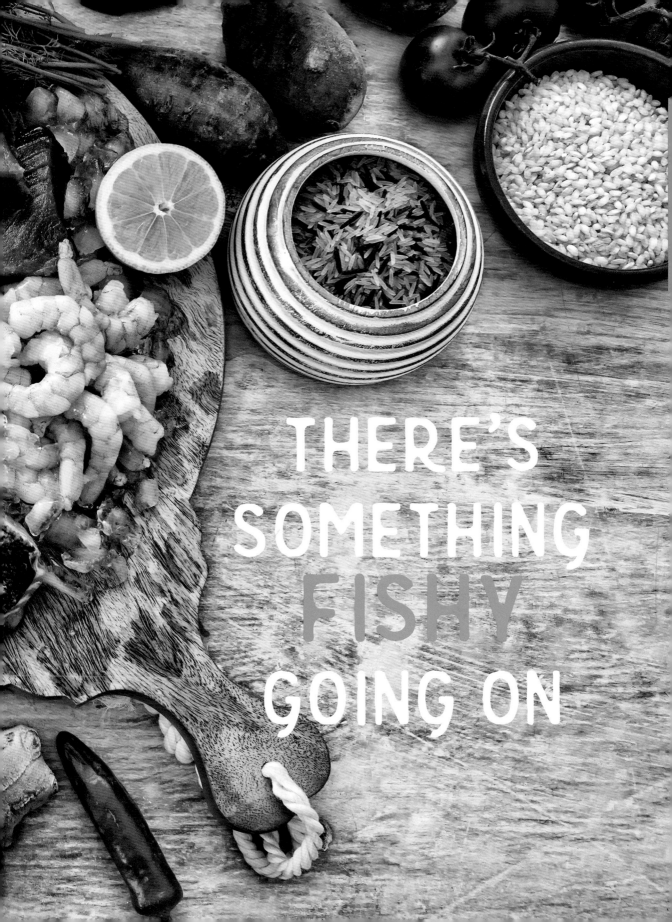

THERE'S SOMETHING FISHY GOING ON

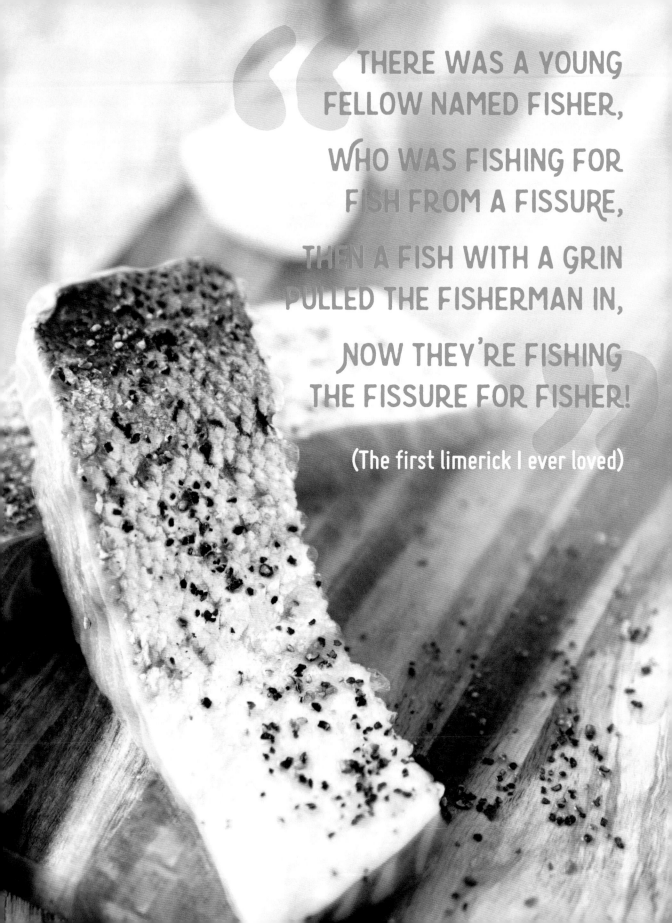

"THERE WAS A YOUNG
FELLOW NAMED FISHER,

WHO WAS FISHING FOR
FISH FROM A FISSURE,

THEN A FISH WITH A GRIN
PULLED THE FISHERMAN IN,

NOW THEY'RE FISHING
THE FISSURE FOR FISHER!"

(The first limerick I ever loved)

OM-E-GA TO TRY THESE DELICIOUS RECIPES!

(IF THAT'S JUST GONE OVER YOUR HEAD, YOU MAY NEED FISH OILS MORE THAN YOU THOUGHT!)

I love fish and fish loves me! For years I suffered severely from the chronic skin condition psoriasis and it was the good fats and oils found in certain fish, along with other foods, that really helped to save the day. Not only is fish good for the skin, but there is now very strong evidence to show that a regular intake of fresh fish can help ward against the Big 3; Heart Disease, Cancer and Stroke.

Fish is a naturally high-protein, low-fat food and white-fleshed fish in particular, is lower in fat than any other source of animal protein. Oily fish are high in omega-3 fatty acids, (the 'good guys' of the 'fat' world) which are extremely important as the body is unable to make significant amounts of these nutrients. This is why 'EFA' stands for essential fatty acids as they are *essential* for our overall health. Evidence suggests that these fats may reduce tissue inflammation and therefore help to alleviate some of the symptoms of rheumatoid arthritis and, in some cases, may also help to reduce depression and mental decline in older people.

As well as being extremely good for you in so many ways, fresh fish also helps to transform otherwise bland dishes into something pretty special. I love a main course raw salad, but add a hot piece of 'melt in your mouth' salmon and BOOM, you've just raised the game substantially. I was a vegan for over four years and the one thing I missed *almost* as much as cheese (well come on!) was my Friday night British staple — Fish 'n' Chips! You'll be pleased to know I have included a healthy version in this section:

* JASEY'S FISH 'N' CHIPS (page 201)
* SWEET CHILLI FISHCAKES WITH A LIME CHILLI & CORIANDER DRESSING (page 157)
* ROASTED MONKFISH RISOTTO, INFUSED WITH FRESH BASIL & LEMON (page 161)

THERE REALLY IS SOMETHING FISHY GOING ON BUT IT'S ALL GOOD!

Remember to snap a pic of whichever fish dish you make and share it on social media to spread the Super *fast* Food message and help to make a difference.

#superfastfood

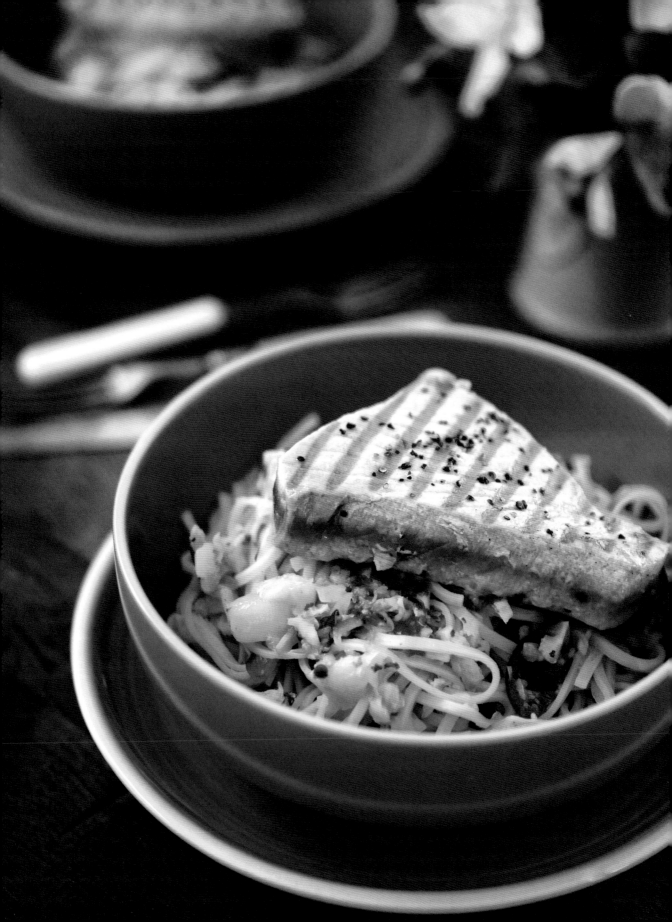

SEARED TUNA ON A BED OF NOODLES WITH A WARM MANGO, ORANGE & CORIANDER SALSA

'You can tuna guitar but you can't tuna fish' was perhaps my favourite joke when I was a wee nipper and although I've grown out of the joke, I'm still a huge fan of the fish. Tuna, when cooked right, is one of those fishes that literally melts in your mouth. It reminds me of fillet steak (back in my red meat eating days), yet the protein in tuna is much easier to digest and is loaded with essential fats. This versatile dish is equally at home come rain or shine. The warm mango and aromatic coriander salsa complements the tuna and noodles beautifully and its deliciously filling too. Enjoy!

INGREDIENTS:

Serves 2

Mango, Orange & Coriander Salsa
Page 241

Olive Oil
1 tablespoon

Ground Black Pepper
1 generous pinch

Tuna Steaks
2 x 150 – 200g/5-7oz steaks

Egg Noodles*
150g/5oz

Boiling Water
1 litre/35fl oz

PREPARE:

Make the Mango, Orange & Coriander Salsa — page 241

Put the olive oil and ground pepper onto a plate, add the tuna steaks and spoon over the oil so both sides of the steaks are covered. Put the noodles into a pan and add the boiling water.

COOK THE NOODLES:

Place the pan of noodles over a low to medium heat and allow to simmer for 5 minutes. Drain the noodles, then add the salsa and noodles back into the warm pan. Toss so all are combined, then place the pan over a low heat for 2 minutes, stirring constantly so that the salsa is warmed through. Then remove from the heat, put the lid on and set to one side.

SEAR THE TUNA:

Place a griddle pan (or you can use a frying pan instead) on the hob over a high heat, when the pan is hot (it will start to smoke a little), place the tuna in the pan and cook on one side for 1.5 – 2 minutes, then turn the tuna over and cook on the other side for a further 1.5 – 2 minutes. Ideally the tuna should still be a little pink in the middle.

SERVE:

Scoop the noodles into a bowl and place the tuna on top.

* If you want this meal to be gluten-free, please use gluten free noodles

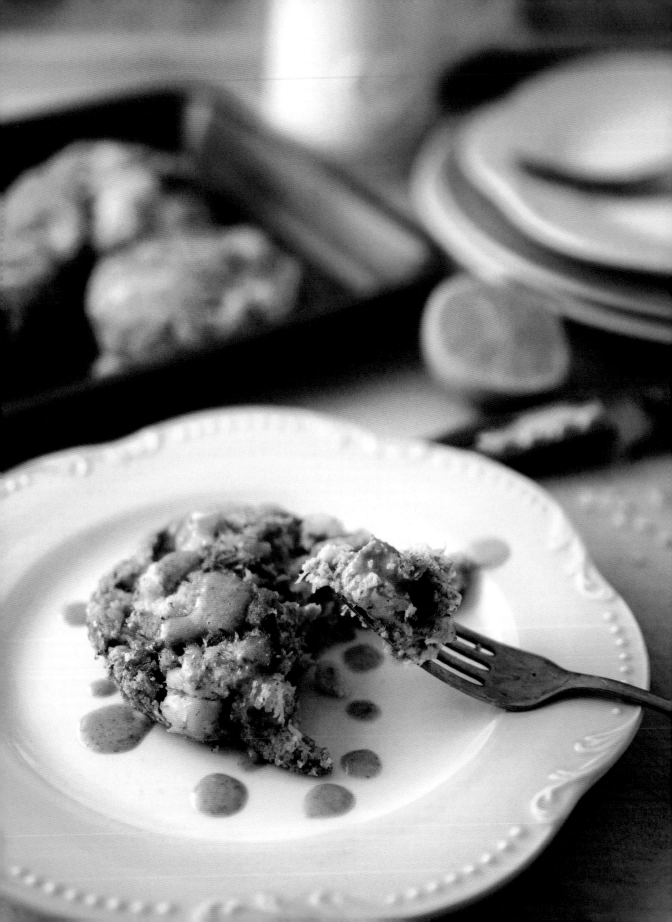

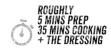

GLUTEN-FREE

CONTAINS NUTS

SWEET CHILLI FISHCAKES WITH A LIME, CHILLI & CORIANDER DRESSING

You can't have a fish section and miss out this classic. These gorgeous, easy-to-make, fishcakes have that chilli kick you want but without blowing your head off. Many times people add too much chilli so it deflects rather than compliments, often to the point where you can't actually enjoy the other ingredients. Serve with a nice fresh side salad and/or a few cheeky sweet potato wedges to make this into a more substantial dish.

INGREDIENTS:

Serves 2

Lime, Chilli & Coriander Dressing
Page 117

Sweet Potato
1 medium

Garlic
2 cloves

Spring Onions
2 sprigs

Red Chilli
1 large

Cod Fillet
200g/7oz (without the skin)

Almonds
100g or 2 handfuls

Olive Oil
1 tablespoon

Himalayan Rock Salt
1 pinch

Ground Black Pepper
1 generous pinch

PREP:

Preheat the oven to 180 °C (350 °F/gas mark 4).

Make the Lime, Chilli & Coriander Dressing — page 117

Peel the sweet potato and chop into chunks. Remove the ends and skin from the garlic. Discard the outer layers and ends from the spring onions and thinly slice. Remove the top and seeds from the red chilli and slice. Chop the cod into small pieces. Using a *Retro Super Blend*, *Bullet* or a hand blender, blitz the almonds for 10 – 20 seconds until they turn into 'flour'.

COOK:

Place the sweet potato and garlic onto a baking tray, drizzle with the olive oil and mix, so all are coated, then place in the oven for 15 minutes stirring part way through.

COMBINE:

Put the cooked sweet potato, garlic, almond 'flour', cod, spring onion, chilli, salt and pepper in a pan (set the baking tray to one side, but do not wash and do not turn the oven off). Mash using a potato masher, so everything is combined but the mixture still contains pieces of fish. Then using your (clean!) hands, divide the mixture into four, shape into 'burgers', then place on the baking tray and pop back in the oven.

COOK:

Cook for 20 minutes.

SERVE:

Gently remove the fishcakes from the tray and either enjoy on their own with the Lime, Chilli & Coriander Dressing, or serve them alongside any of the salads found on pages 81–107.

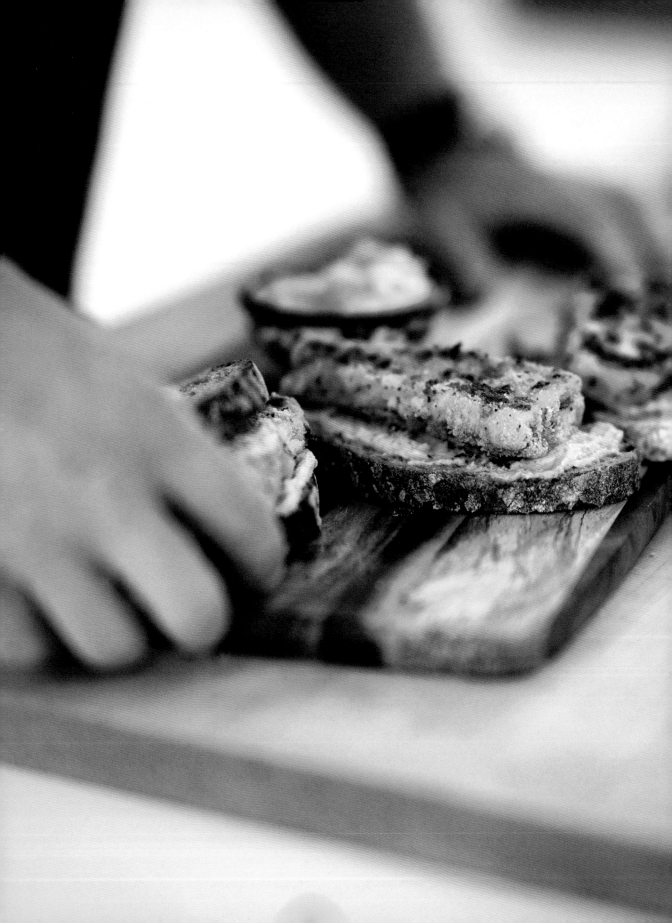

JASEY'S BAD BOY FISH FINGER SANDWICH WITH A CHEEKY, TANGY, DAIRY-FREE AVO TARTAR!

There are fish finger sandwiches and then there's this bad boy. Fish finger sandwiches remind me of my childhood, as they were a regular feature in the Vale household at least once a week. Back then of course, it was shop bought 'fish' fingers, slapped between two bits of white bread and loaded with butter and shop bought tartar sauce. These days the focus is still on taste, but also on making sure it gets a good nod in the health direction too. Beautiful fresh fish, coated in spelt flour, breadcrumbs and chives and served between two slices of wholesome bread which have been generously smothered in a creamy, fresh, homemade avocado tartar. **ENJOY!**

INGREDIENTS:

Serves 2

FOR THE TANGY AVO TARTAR:

White Onion
½
Ripe Avocado
½ medium
Lemon
½ (the juice of)
Dijon Mustard
2 heaped teaspoons
Cider Vinegar
1 tablespoon
Capers
1 heaped tablespoon

FOR THE FISH FINGERS:

Vietnamese River Cobbler Fish
(or any other white fish)
250g/9 oz
Spelt Rye Flour
4 tablespoons
Himalayan Rock Salt
1 pinch
Ground Black Pepper
1 pinch
Egg (free-range organic)
1 medium
Chives
10g or 1 small handful
Breadcrumbs
80g /3 oz
Olive Oil
1 tablespoon
Good Quality Bread
(sourdough is recommended) 4 slices

PREPARE:

Peel and dice the onion, remove the avocado flesh (discard the skin and stone). Cut the fish into four even 'fish finger' shaped pieces and put to one side.

BLEND:

Place the onion, avocado, lemon juice, mustard, vinegar and capers in the small container of a hand blender or *Retro Super Blend*. Pulse for 10 – 20 seconds, so it is creamy but still has a rough texture. Then place in the fridge.

PREPARE:

Place the spelt rye flour, salt and pepper into a mixing bowl. Whisk the egg and pour into a shallow bowl. Finely chop the chives and place in a separate shallow bowl along with the breadcrumbs.

CREATE:

Coat the fish in the flour, then in the egg wash and finally into the breadcrumbs, making sure the ends are coated.

COOK:

Place the olive oil in the frying pan and then cook the fish over a medium to high heat for 3 – 4 minutes each side and finish by turning the heat up high for 20 seconds each side.

ASSEMBLE:

Use the tartar as 'butter' and spread over each slice of bread, then create your fish finger sandwich!

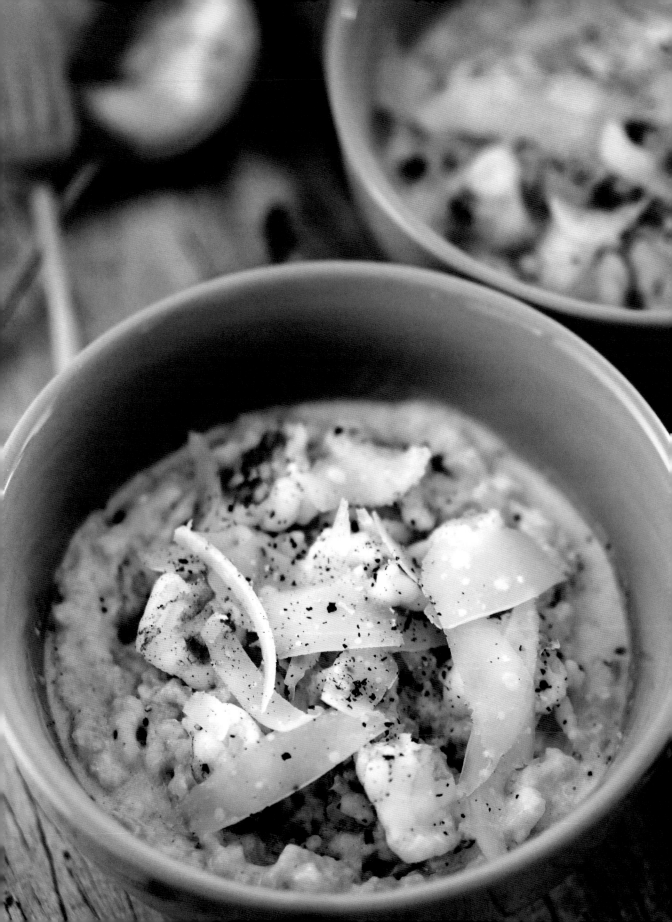

ROASTED MONKFISH RISOTTO, INFUSED WITH FRESH BASIL & LEMON

GLUTEN-FREE

YOU MUST MAKE THIS ONE! Yes, it's me shouting again, but when you taste this you'll be pleased I did. This recipe book wasn't designed to be simply flicked through to look at the nice pictures! I could bang on about the nutrient content of this dish, and it's a winner clearly on that front, but the real magic is in the taste. I won't say anymore, just make it, savour it and close your eyes on the first bite to make sure you capture the essence of one of my favourite recipes of all time.

INGREDIENTS:

Serves 2

Red Onion
½ medium

Garlic
2 cloves

Parmesan or Parmigiano Reggiano Cheese
50g/2oz

Monkfish
300g/11oz

Olive Oil
5 tablespoons

Fresh Basil
30g or 1 handful

Lemon (the juice of)
1

Stock Cube
1

Boiling Water
500ml/17.5fl oz

Risotto
200g/7oz

Crème Fraîche
50ml/2fl oz

Ground Black Pepper
2 generous pinches

Himalayan Rock Salt
1 pinch

PREPARE:

Remove the ends and skin from the onion and garlic and dice. Using a vegetable peeler, slice ¼ of the cheese into thin slices and roughly chop the other ¾. Remove any bones from the monkfish and cut into bite sized pieces. Pat the monkfish with kitchen roll to absorb as much water as possible (this will make sure it browns when cooking and doesn't just boil in its own juices!). Place the monkfish on a small plate and drizzle 1 tablespoon of olive oil over the fish, making sure all sides are coated.

Place the basil, 3 tablespoons of olive oil, the lemon juice and the roughly chopped cheese into the container of a hand blender or *Retro Super Blend / Bullet* and blitz for 30 seconds. Dissolve the stock cube in the boiling water.

COOK:

Place the remaining olive oil in a large pan and place on the hob over a medium to high heat. Add the onion and garlic and cook for 5 minutes stirring frequently. Add the risotto and cook for 2 minutes, stirring constantly. Add ¼ of the stock, reduce the heat and allow most of the liquid to absorb, then repeat the process until all the liquid has been gradually added and absorbed (stirring intermittently). Add the basil/ oil/lemon/cheese mix, the crème fraîche, 1 pinch of pepper and the salt. Stir well, remove from the heat, cover with the lid and set to one side.

FINALLY:

Heat a griddle pan over a high heat, then add the monkfish and cook for 2 minutes each side.

SERVE:

Spoon the risotto into a shallow bowl, add the monkfish and finish with the remaining black pepper and cheese.

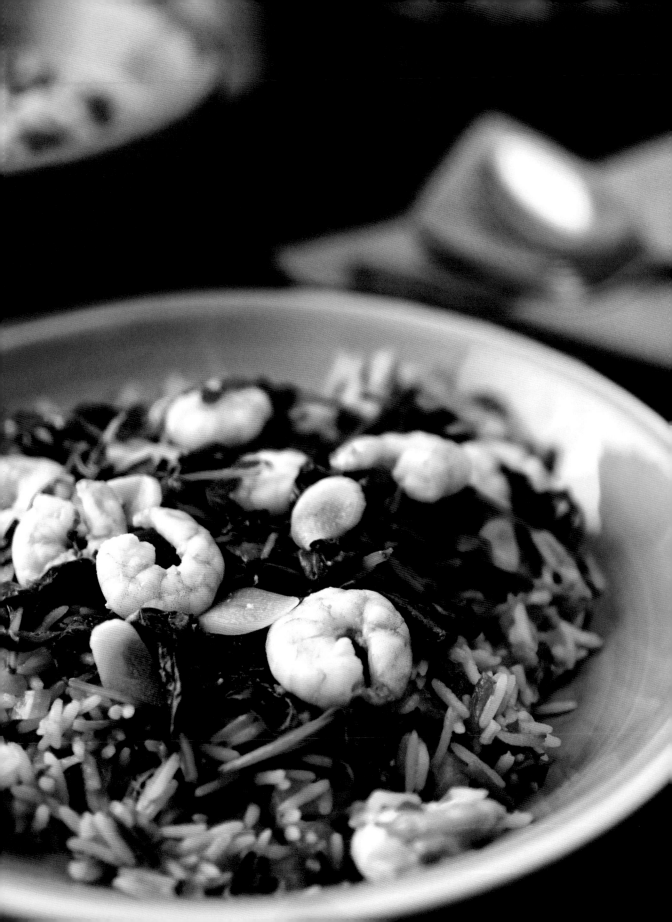

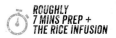

GLUTEN-FREE

PAN FRIED CHILLI & GARLIC KING PRAWNS WITH A RICH TOMATO & WILD RICE INFUSION

There's something about king prawns cooked in chilli and garlic that hits the spot every time. This recipe is rich in protein, fibre, vitamins, minerals, antioxidants, natural healers and, according to Chinese medicine, it can delay the onset of aging, dementia and even prolong sexual libido! Well, not this specific recipe clearly, but rather the prawns. Prawns are said to be good for the kidneys and Chinese medicine believes the strength and weakness of a male's sexual libido, has an enormous direct correlation with the strength and weakness of the kidneys. Therefore, those with poor kidney function should frequently consume prawns, and those who frequently eat prawns, can delay the onset of aging, dementia and prolong sexual libido. Right, where's the pan!

INGREDIENTS:

Serves 2

Rich Tomato & Wild Rice Infusion
Page 233
Chillies
2 Medium
Garlic
2 cloves
Lime
1/2
Sesame Oil
1 tablespoon
King Prawns (uncooked)
200g/7 oz
Baby Leaf Spinach
100g or 2 large handfuls

PREPARE:

Make the Tomato & Wild Rice Infusion — page 233

Cut the chillies in half, remove the tops and slice. Remove any hard ends from the garlic, peel and finely slice. Cut the lime in half.

COOK:

Add the oil to a wok (or frying pan) and place over a medium to high heat. Add the garlic and chilli and cook for 2 minutes. Then add the king prawns, and spinach and cook for a further 3 minutes, stirring frequently to ensure all the prawns are cooked (they will turn pink).

SERVE:

Pile a generous serving of the Rich Tomato & Wild Rice Infusion into a bowl, add the pan-fried prawns and serve with the chunk of lime.

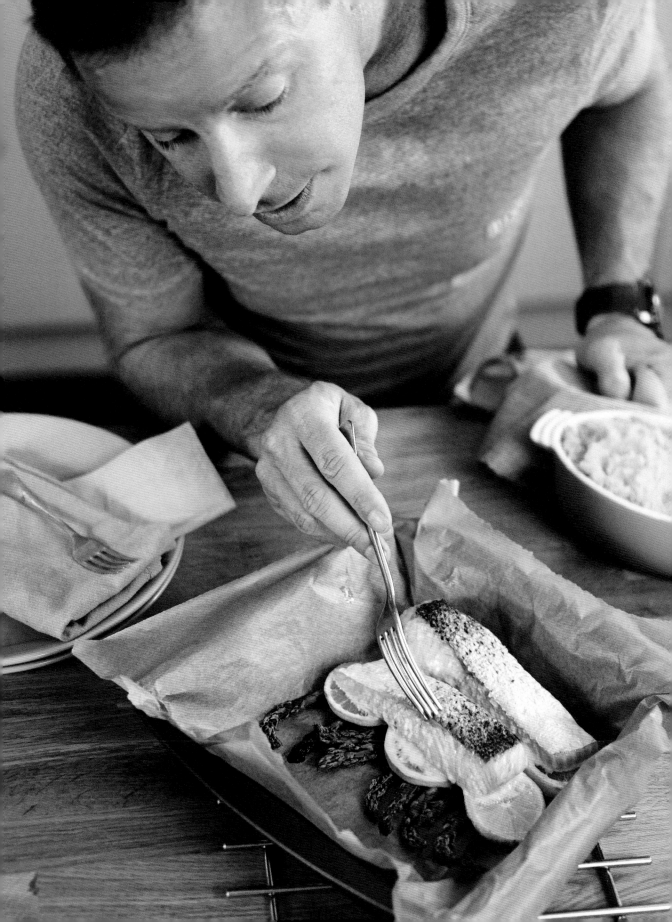

SALMON 'N' SWEET POTATO, GARLIC & PARMESAN MASH

GLUTEN-FREE

There are very few things, on the food side of life that I like more than fresh salmon. In fact, there are times when my entire meal will consist of just a nice large piece of freshly cooked salmon that just melts in your mouth. However, place this genuine superfood on top of some creamy, Sweet Potato Garlic & Parmesan Mash and the already wonderful is transported to another dimension. This dish is so ridiculously easy to make that it's well at home in the 'almost effortless' camp. If you are throwing dinner for a few friends and want to actually enjoy their company (rather than spending all your time in the kitchen), then this dish is perfect for such an occasion. Beautifully satisfying, wonderfully filling and nutritionally sound — BOOM!

INGREDIENTS:

Serves 2

Sweet Potato, Garlic & Parmesan Mash
Page 231

Asparagus
150g/5oz

Lemon
1

Salmon (with the skin on)
2 x 130g — 150g/4–5oz fillets

Olive Oil
1 tablespoon

Himalayan Rock Salt
1 pinch

PREPARE:

Preheat the oven to 200 °C (400 °F/gas mark 6).

Make the Sweet Potato, Garlic & Parmesan Mash — page 231

Cut the hard ends off the asparagus. Cut the lemon into slices (discarding the ends). Line a baking tray with a sheet of greaseproof paper and lay the asparagus on top, then lay the sliced lemon over the asparagus. Rest the salmon on top of the lemon (skin side up) and drizzle with the olive oil before sprinkling with the salt.

COOK:

Place the baking tray in the oven and cook for 20 minutes.

SERVE:

Put the salmon and asparagus on top of the lovely mash.

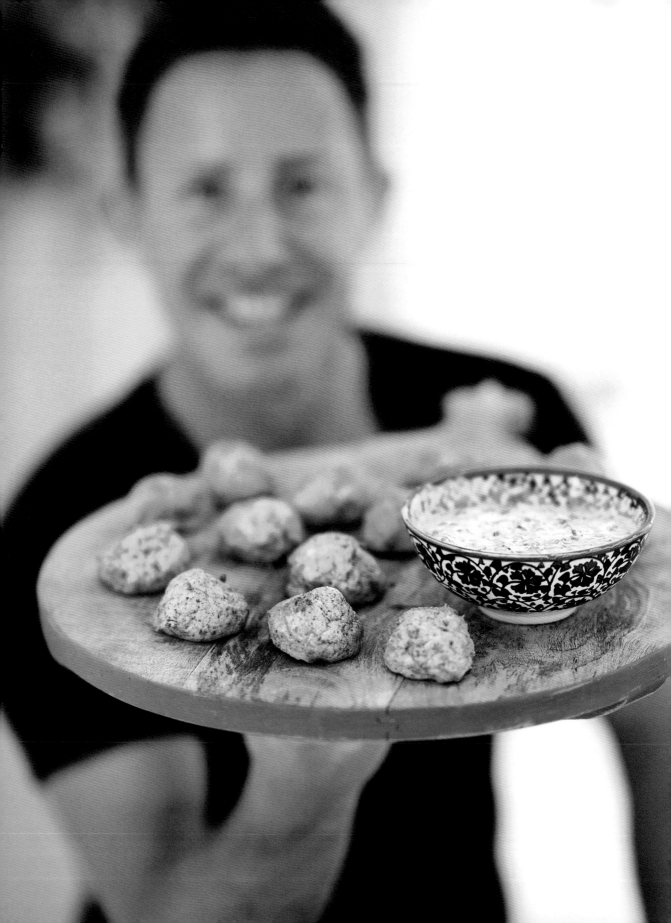

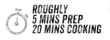
GREAT 'FISH BALLS' OF FIRE WITH A CREAMY GARLIC & CHIVE BLAST

GLUTEN-FREE

Every time I bite into one of these beauties all I can hear are the wonderful tones of rock 'n' roll legend Jerry Lee Lewis, "Goodness, gracious, great balls of fire" — well, great 'fish balls' of fire to be precise! It's the chilli in the balls themselves and the pungent touch of garlic in the yogurt and chive blast, that creates the fire. But don't panic, as the cooling yogurt acts as the perfect ying to the fiery yang. This recipe makes an average of sixteen fish balls, so more than enough for two as a stand-alone meal. However, these little babies also work particularly well as canapés if hosting a Super *fast* Food dinner party!

INGREDIENTS:

Serves 2

FOR THE FISH BALLS:

Olive Oil
2 teaspoons
Chillies
2 medium
Salmon (skinless and boneless)
500g/17.5 oz
Pumpkin Seeds
100g/3.5 oz
Organic Free-Range Egg
1
Himalayan Rock Salt
1 pinch
Ground Black Pepper
1 pinch

FOR THE CREAMY GARLIC & CHIVE BLAST:

Garlic
2 cloves
Chives
20g or 1 small handful
Spring Onions
2
Cucumber
50g or 3 cm
Lemon
½ (the juice of)
Yogurt
4 tablespoons
Himalayan Rock Salt
1 pinch

PREPARE THE BALLS:

Preheat the oven to 170 °C (340 °F / gas mark 4).

Line a baking tin with greaseproof paper and cover with the olive oil.

CREATE THE BALLS:

Remove the ends from the chillies and dice (do not remove the seeds). Dice the salmon. Grind the pumpkin seeds into a 'flour' using a hand blender or *Retro Super Blend / Bullet*, then add all the other ingredients for the fish balls. Pulse until all are combined. Then, using 2 tablespoons, mould the mixture into even sized balls and place on the oiled greaseproof paper.

COOK:

Pop the baking tray in the oven for 20 minutes.

MEANWHILE PREPARE THE DRESSING:

Peel the garlic. Finely chop the chives, spring onion, cucumber and garlic. Place all the ingredients for the dressing in a bowl and gently combine.

ASSEMBLE:

Once the balls are cooked, serve with a very generous scoop of the Garlic & Chive Blast.

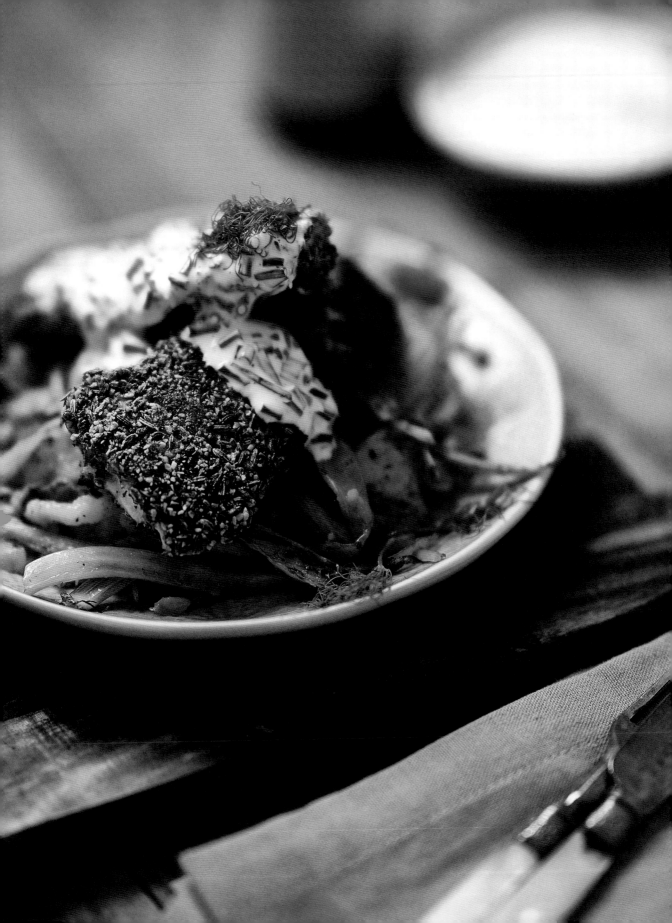

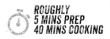

GLUTEN-FREE

FISH FILLET WITH A FENNEL SEED CRUST
SERVED ON A BED OF SMASHED NEW POTATOES, WILTED FENNEL AND FINISHED WITH A LEMON & CHIVE INFUSED CRÈME FRAÎCHE

If you're wondering whether the taste of this recipe can possibly live up to the descriptive power above, the simple answer is YES! The highlight has to be the fennel seed crust, and once combined with the succulent fish and cheeky scoop of crème fraîche, it will rock your taste bud boat quite beautifully. So, why not organise a little dinner party as it's time to impress the hell out of your friends!

INGREDIENTS:

Serves 2

Olive Oil
4 tablespoons
New Potatoes
500g/17.5 oz
Himalayan Rock Salt
2 generous pinches
Ground Black Pepper
2 generous pinches
Chives
15g or 1 small handful
Crème Fraîche
100ml/3.5 fl oz
Lemon
½ (the juice of)
Fennel Bulb
300g/10oz
Pumpkin Seeds
30g/1 oz
Fennel Seeds
15g/0.5 oz
Free-Range Organic Egg
1
Vietnamese River Cobbler Fish
(or any other white fish)
250g/9 oz

PREPARE:

Preheat the oven to 180 °C (350 °F / gas mark 4)
Place 1 tablespoon of olive oil into the baking tray and pop in the oven to warm. Cut the new potatoes in pieces roughly 2–3 cm in size, then place in the warmed baking tray with 1 pinch of salt and pepper. Give the tray a good shake to coat the potatoes and pop in the oven for 25 minutes. Finely chop the chives. Place the crème fraîche in a small bowl, add the lemon juice and chives, mix well and pop in the fridge. Remove the hard end from the fennel and thinly slice.

WILT:

Place 1 tablespoon of olive oil in a large saucepan over a medium to high heat, add the sliced fennel and allow to cook for 10 — 15 minutes, stirring occasionally.

MEANWHILE:

Place the pumpkin and fennel seeds in the small container of a hand blender or *Retro Super Blend* and grind for a few seconds until they form a 'flour'. Whisk the egg in a shallow bowl.

LET'S GET FISHY:

Cut the fish into four pieces. Place the ground seeds on a plate. Dip the fish into the bowl of egg and then onto the plate of ground seeds, ensuring all sides are covered with the seed blend.

COOK:

Place 1 tablespoon of olive oil in a frying pan and heat over a medium heat. Add the coated fish and cook on each side for 3 minutes.

MEANWHILE:

Add the final tablespoon of olive oil, salt and pepper to the pan of fennel and then add the new potatoes. Using a potato masher gently squash some of the potatoes and mix well with a wooden spoon.

COOK:

Place the smashed potatoes and fennel in the centre of a plate, pop the fish on top and finish with a generous dollop of the Infused Crème Fraîche.

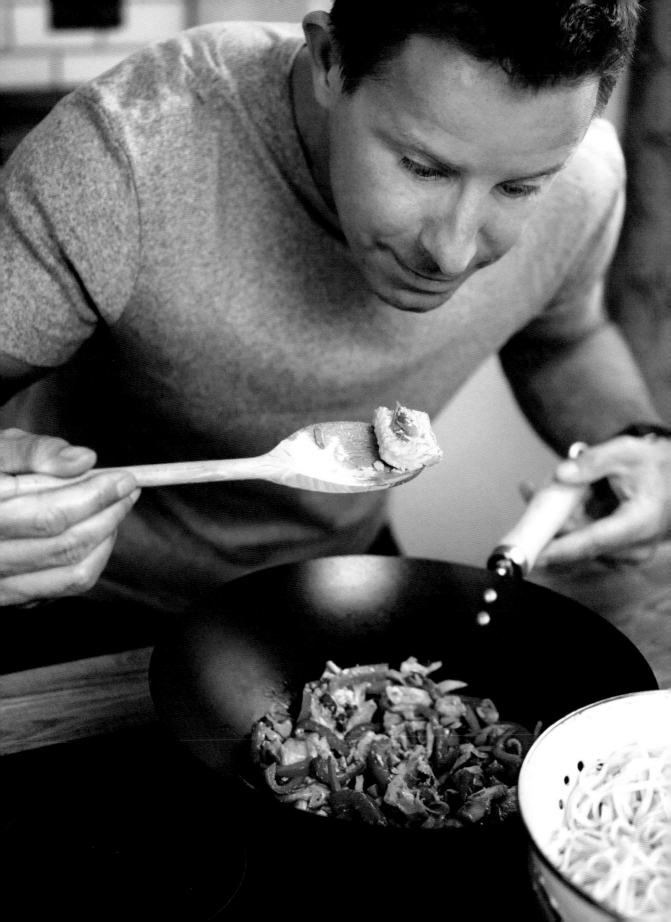

SALMON MARINATED IN SOY SAUCE, GINGER, CHILLI & HONEY, SERVED WITH SPRING ONIONS, RED PEPPER & EGG NOODLES

This dish works best with a little pre-planning. So allow about an hour or more before you are ready to eat, to prepare the salmon in the marinade and leave in the fridge to really help all those wonderful flavours to infuse. This dish has an obvious oriental feel to it and is light, slightly fiery, incredibly healthy and tastes amazing.

INGREDIENTS FOR THE MARINADE:

Serves 2

Fresh Ginger
30g or 2 cm x 4 cm

Red Chilli
1 medium

Salmon Fillets (skinless)
2 x 150g/5oz

Soy Sauce
2 tablespoons

Honey
1 tablespoon

INGREDIENTS FOR THE NOODLES:

Spring Onions
2 sprigs

Red Pepper
1 medium

Coconut Oil
1 tablespoon

Egg Noodles
150g/5oz

Boiling Water
1 litre/35fl oz

TO PREPARE THE SALMON:

Peel the ginger and slice into matchstick sized pieces. Remove the top from the chilli, cut in half and thinly slice. Cut the salmon into bite sized pieces. Put the soy sauce, honey, ginger and chilli into a small mixing bowl and mix until all the honey is combined. Add the salmon, spoon over the marinade, cover with cling film and place in the fridge for at least 20 minutes or for best results 1 — 2 hours.

TO PREPARE THE NOODLES:

Remove the ends and outer skin from the spring onions and slice diagonally. Cut the red pepper into quarters; remove the core and seeds and slice.

COOK:

Put the coconut oil in a wok (or frying pan) and warm on a medium heat, then add the spring onions, peppers, salmon, ginger and chilli (retaining most of the marinade in the mixing bowl). Turn the salmon pieces so they sear on both sides and allow to cook for 4 – 6 minutes.

MEANWHILE...

Place the noodles and boiling water into a saucepan and boil for 3 minutes, then drain, return the noodles to the warm pan, pour over the marinade, stir so all the noodles are coated and cover with the lid.

SERVE:

Place the noodles directly onto the plate, and top with the salmon and veggies.

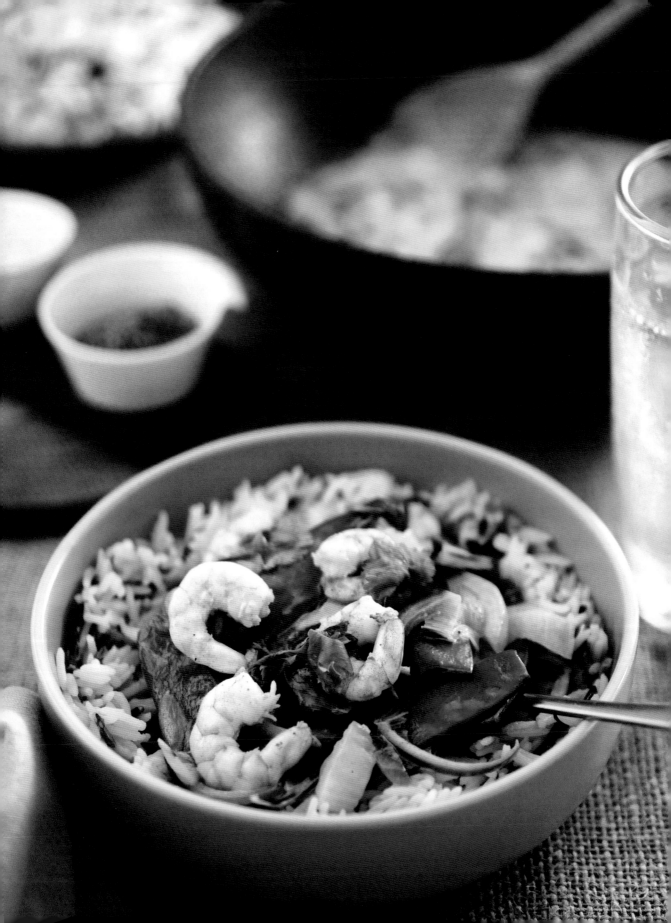

GLUTEN-FREE

KING PRAWN & COCONUT CURRY WITH GARLIC FRIED RICE

If you like curry, you'll LOVE this. Again, genuinely easy to make and hits all the nutritional buttons you'd expect. Prawns, garlic, mange tout, red onion, bell pepper and coconut milk can all be described as superfoods, supplying the body and mind with an impressive display of the essential nutrients required for optimum health.

INGREDIENTS FOR THE CURRY:

Serves 2

Ground Cumin
1 teaspoon

Cayenne Pepper
½ teaspoon

Nutmeg
½ teaspoon

Coconut Oil
1 tablespoon

Red Onion
½ medium

Yellow Pepper
1 medium

Mange Tout
75g or 1 large handful

Pak Choi
1 medium bulb

Fresh Coriander
30g or 1 handful

Coconut Milk
400ml/14fl oz or 1 can

King Prawns (uncooked)
200g/7 oz

INGREDIENTS FOR THE RICE:

Red Onion
½ medium

Garlic
3 cloves

Basmati Rice
150g/5oz

Boiling Water
450ml/16fl oz

Coconut Oil
1 tablespoon

Himalayan Rock Salt
1 generous pinch

PREPARE THE CURRY:

Place the cumin, cayenne pepper, nutmeg and 1 tablespoon of coconut oil in a small bowl and mix. Remove the end from the onion, peel, cut in half and finely slice. Cut the yellow pepper in half, remove the core and seeds and thinly slice. Remove the ends and any stringy spines from the mange tout. Remove the end from the pak choi and slice. Coarsely chop the coriander.

PREPARE THE RICE:

Remove the end from the onion, peel and finely dice. Peel the garlic, crush with the back of a knife and chop into small pieces. Rinse the basmati rice, place in a pan and add the boiling water.

BOIL:

Place the pan with the rice over a high heat and bring to the boil, cover with the lid, reduce the heat and allow to simmer for 20 – 25 minutes, until all the water has been absorbed. Keep an eye on the rice and add a little more water if needed.

MEANWHILE...

Place 1 tablespoon of coconut oil in a large pan over a medium to high heat, then add the diced onion and garlic and allow to cook for 5 minutes. Once the rice is cooked, remove from heat, drain any excess water and add to the onions and garlic. Add the salt, stir well and cook for 2 — 3 minutes, then remove from the heat and cover with a lid.

COOK THE CURRY:

Put the oil and spices in a wok or frying pan and place over a medium heat. Add the red onion, yellow pepper, mange tout, and allow to cook for 5 minutes stirring occasionally. Then add the pak choi, coriander, coconut milk and prawns, bring to the boil and then reduce the heat and allow to simmer for 5 minutes.

SERVE:

Place the rice into a shallow bowl and spoon over the curry.

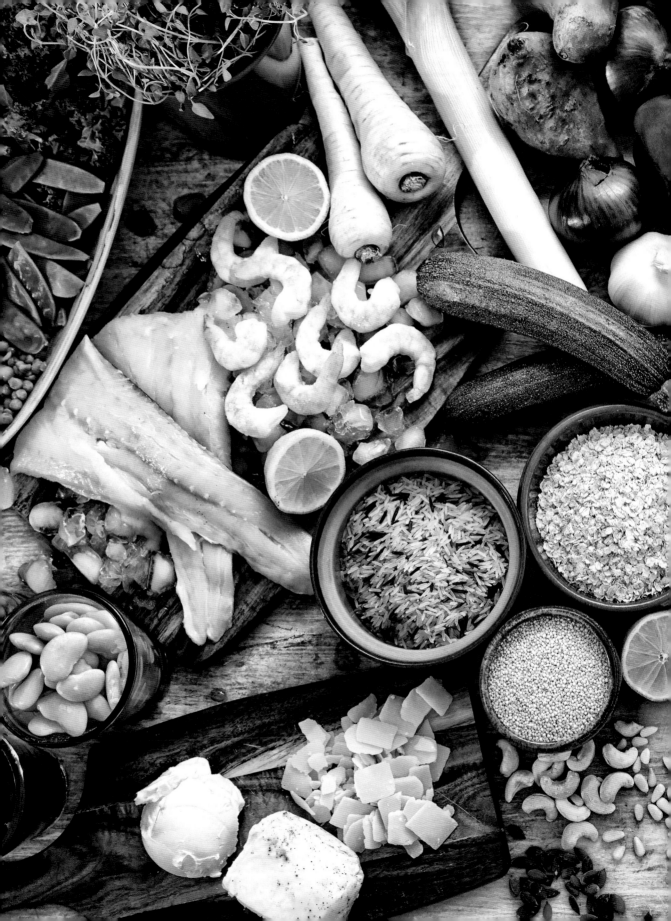

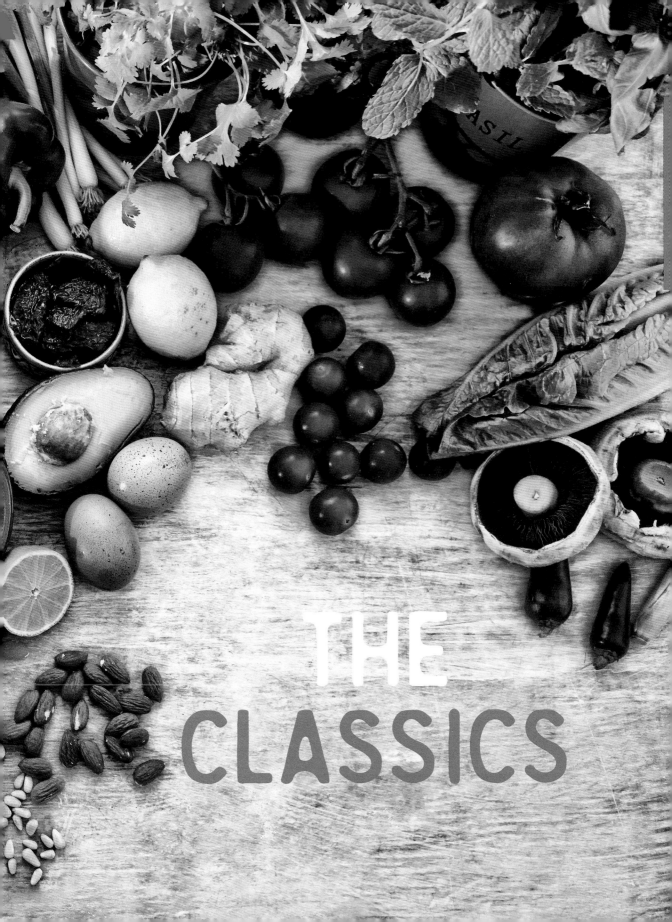

THE
CLASSICS

THE DOCTOR OF THE FUTURE WILL NO LONGER TREAT THE HUMAN FRAME WITH DRUGS, BUT RATHER WILL CURE AND PREVENT DISEASE WITH NUTRITION

THOMAS EDISON

CLASSIC DISHES WITH A HEALTHY TWIST

I have a sneaky feeling that there will be more recipes made from this section of the book than any other. I think it's fair to say that the reason a **dish gets 'classic' status**, is because it's extremely popular. In other words, it's **because most people love it**. One of the fears a lot of people have when switching to a healthier way of eating is that they will have to say goodbye to their favorite comforting, classic dishes. However, there isn't a single classic dish that cannot be 'healthified' – if there is such a word (there isn't so please don't look it up!)

By simply getting smart with ingredients, you can get all of the texture and flavor of a classic without the portion of obesity and ill health on the side! If, for example, you love burgers and fries but feel a veggie burger could never get close to its meaty rival, why not knock up my **Spicy Mint 'n' Avo Veggie Burger** (page 179) with a side of **Sweet Chilli Potato Wedges** (page 211) and I guarantee it will be a game changer for you. If you are more of a pizza person but think you cannot make a pizza without the dough, then you must tuck into my **'No Dough' Halloumi, Basil & Pine Nut Pizza** (page 197) and prepare yourself to be blown away.

You'll also find:

* VEGGIE BANGERS 'N' MASH WITH RED ONION GRAVY (page 185)
* SUPER-PIMPED, SUPERFOOD CAESAR (page 189)
* NO SHEEP SHEPHERD'S PIE! (page 191)

Other than the **Super Salads**, this is my favorite section of the book and on a cold winters eve, a classic of some kind usually gets it! I also love this section because even if you are the only health conscious person in your household, you won't get anyone turning their nose up at these dishes, so no need to make one meal for you and one for them! **These really are 'comfort food' classics made healthy**, all loaded with pure nutrition and all bursting with flavor.

Remember to snap a pic of whichever classic dish takes your fancy and share it on social media to spread the **Super *fast* Food** message and help to make a difference.

#superfastfood

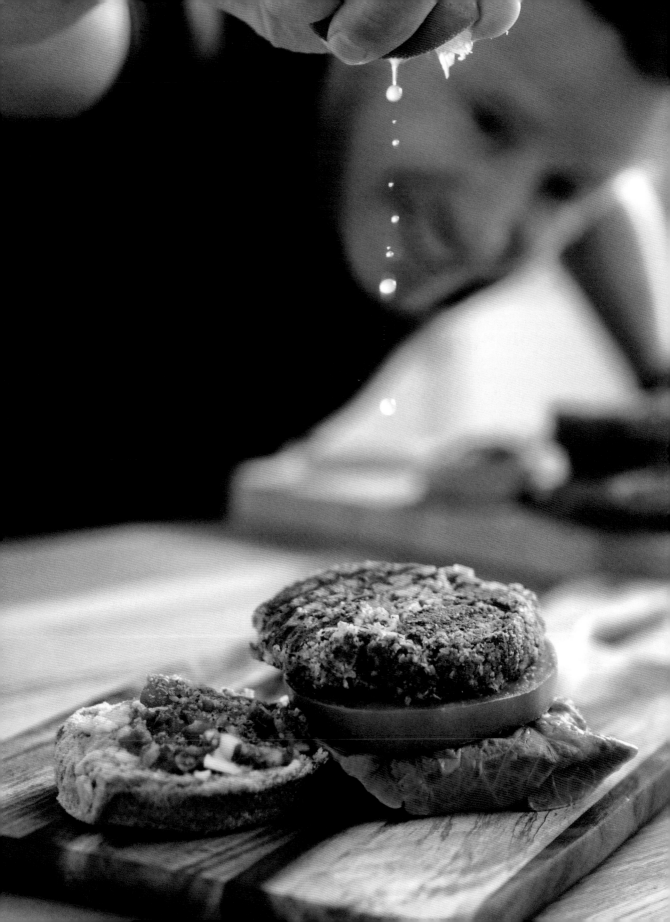

JASEY'S SPICY MINT 'N' AVO VEGGIE BURGER

There are veggie burgers and then there's this bad boy! Sometimes words just aren't enough and this is one such occasion. I used to be a burger, fries and apple pie boy, one of the many things that lead to me being fat and ill. I thought my burger days were long gone, but this extremely healthy veggie burger tastes even better than the real thing (in my humble opinion) and you can eat it guilt free — so put that in your bun and eat it! Great on its own, even better with some sweet potato fries on the side.

GLUTEN-FREE

VEGAN

VEGETARIAN

CONTAINS NUTS

INGREDIENTS:

Serves 2

Almonds
40g or 1 handful

Sunflower Seeds
1 tablespoon

Pumpkin Seeds
1 tablespoon

Peas (fresh or frozen)
100g/3.5oz

Butter Beans (canned)
100g/3.5oz

Fresh Mint
30g or 1 Large Handful

Ground Cumin
1 pinch

Cayenne Pepper
1 pinch

Himalayan Rock Salt
1 pinch

Olive Oil
1 tablespoon

Avocado (ripe)
½

Gluten Free Buns
2 (optional 'no bun' burger)

Beef Tomato
1

Romaine Lettuce
1 small

Ground Black Pepper
1 pinch

Lime (the juice of)
1

Wooden Skewer
2

PREPARE:

Put the almonds, sunflower and pumpkin seeds in a food processor and blitz until they turn into 'flour'. Keep a handful of the 'flour' to one side to coat the finished burgers. Put the peas, butter beans, mint, cumin, cayenne pepper, salt and the remaining 'flour' into the food processor and blend.

SHAPE:

Divide the mixture in half and using your (clean!) hands make into two burgers. Place the reserved 'flour' on a chopping board or plate, lay the burgers on top and lightly coat both sides.

FREEZE:

Place in the freezer for 10 minutes to firm.

HEAT:

Put the oil in a frying pan and place over a medium heat. Add the burgers and cook for 6 minutes on each side.

MEANWHILE...

If using a bun, spread the avocado flesh like 'butter' on the buns, if going for the 'no bun' option, simply slice the avocado. Cut the beef tomato so you have two good size slices.

SERVE:

Arrange your burger or 'no bun' burger in any way you chose using the tomato, lettuce, avocado and burger. Add a pinch of ground black pepper and a squeeze of lime. Push a wooden skewer through the middle and BOOM, your burger is done!

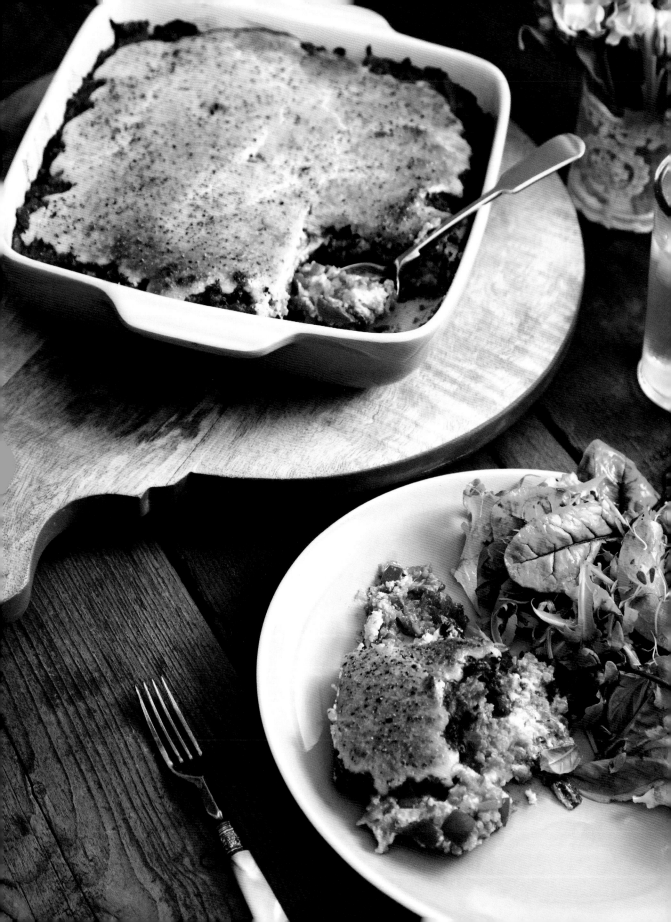

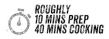

VEGGIE LAYERED LASAGNE

When you taste this lasagne you'll be convinced it contains meat. This is because I have added quinoa to the tomato sauce to thicken it up and give it a 'meaty' texture. This healthy version is gluten-free, tastes amazing and is super fast to make compared to traditional Lasagne.

GLUTEN-FREE

VEGAN

VEGETARIAN

CONTAINS NUTS

INGREDIENTS FOR THE CHEESE SAUCE

Serves 2

Cashew Nuts
100g or 2 large handfuls
Filtered Water
60ml/2fl oz
Goats Cheese* (soft)
100g/3.5oz
Mustard
1 flat teaspoon
Himalayan Rock Salt
1 pinch

PREP:

Preheat the oven to 220 °C (450 °F/gas mark 7).

PREP FOR THE CHEESE SAUCE:

Put the cashew nuts in the container of a hand blender and blitz for 10 — 20 seconds until they turn into 'flour' (leave in the container).

PREP FOR THE TOMATO SAUCE:

Remove the ends, peel and finely dice the onion and garlic. Finely chop the fresh and sun-dried tomatoes. Remove the core and seeds from the red pepper and finely chop. Roughly chop the basil, discarding any hard stems. Dissolve the stock cube in the boiling water.

MAKE THE TOMATO SAUCE:

Heat the oil over a medium to high heat, add the onion and garlic and cook for 5 minutes or until soft. Add the tomatoes, peppers, vinegar, quinoa, basil, cayenne pepper, salt and stock. Stir well, then reduce to a medium heat, cover with the lid and allow to simmer for 20 minutes, stirring occasionally. Remove the lid and allow to cook for a further 5 minutes so the sauce thickens (stirring frequently).

MEANWHILE... PREPARE THE LAYERS:

- Remove the ends from the courgettes and cut lengthways into thin slices (about 0.5 cm thick). Place the courgette in a dish and drizzle with the olive oil, turning so all are coated.

* If vegan, replace with 4 tablespoons of nutritional yeast or simply leave the cheese out.

INGREDIENTS FOR THE 'TOMATO SAUCE' AND 'THE LAYERS' ON THE NEXT PAGE ⧸⧸⧸●——→

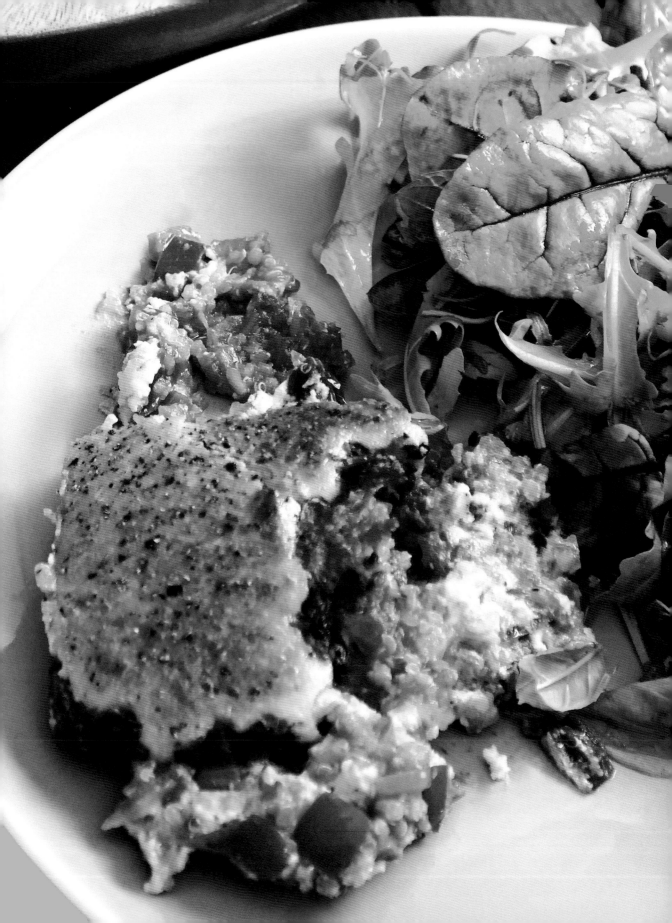

VEGGIE LAYERED LASAGNE (CONTINUED)

GLUTEN-FREE

VEGAN

VEGETARIAN

CONTAINS NUTS

INGREDIENTS FOR THE TOMATO SAUCE:

Red Onion
½ medium

Garlic
2 cloves

Fresh Tomatoes
6 medium

Sun-Dried Tomatoes
150g/5oz

Red Pepper
1 medium

Fresh Basil
20g or 1 handful

Stock Cube
1

Boiling Water
120ml/4fl oz

Olive Oil
1 tablespoon

Apple Cider Vinegar
1 tablespoon

Quinoa (or Bulgur wheat)
40g/1.5oz

Cayenne Pepper
1 pinch

Himalayan Rock Salt
1 generous pinch

INGREDIENTS FOR THE LAYERS:

Courgettes / Zucchinis
2 medium

Olive Oil
1 tablespoon

Ground Black Pepper
4 pinches

GRIDDLE:

Heat a griddle or frying pan and cook the courgette strips over a high heat, turning regularly until they are cooked on both sides (you will need to do this in batches). If these are ready before the sauce, just allow to cool.

MEANWHILE... MAKE THE CHEESE SAUCE:

Add the filtered water, goats cheese, mustard and salt to the cashew 'flour' in the hand blender container and blitz for 10 — 20 seconds until it forms a smooth sauce.

ASSEMBLE:

Place a layer of courgette on the bottom of the baking dish (cut to size if needed). Next create a second layer using half of the tomato sauce, followed by a third layer using half of the cheese sauce. Repeat with the remaining ingredients and finish with the ground black pepper.

COOK:

Pop in the oven and cook for 15 minutes or until the lasagne starts to brown.

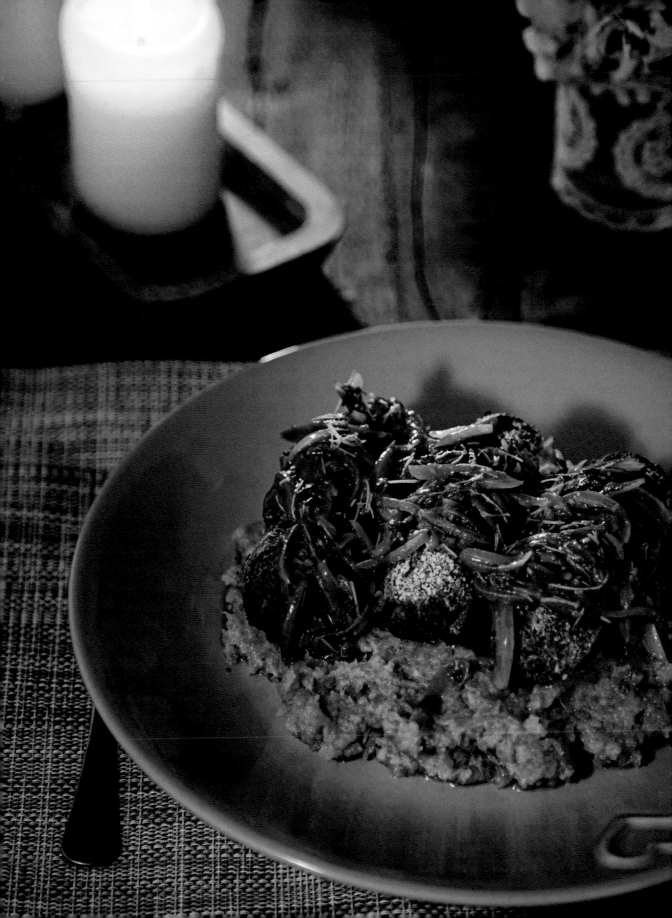

GLUTEN-FREE

VEGAN

VEGETARIAN

CONTAINS NUTS

VEGGIE BANGERS 'N' MASH WITH RED ONION GRAVY

You can't have a 'classic' section without including this true British classic. I have always loved bangers and mash but since leaving 'mystery food' behind (what's in the average meat sausage? Exactly, it's a mystery!) I had to find another way of getting the wonderful classic tastes of this dish. Now making a good veggie sausage isn't as easy as it may appear and it took me a while to get this right. What I will say is, if making your own veggie sausages feels like a little too much faff for you, feel free to go and grab some good ready-made ones. Whatever route you go for, a good veggie sausage on a bed of sweet potato mash with some
red onion gravy is one classic you won't want to miss.

INGREDIENTS:

Serves 2

Olive Oil for the baking tray
½ tablespoon

INGREDIENTS FOR THE BANGERS:

Almonds
60g or 1 large handful
Pumpkin Seeds
40g or 1 handful
Himalayan Rock Salt
2 pinches
Ground Black Pepper
2 generous pinches
Leek
1 small
Garlic
2 cloves
Mushrooms
4 medium
Baking Apple
1 small
Olive Oil
1 tablespoon
Dijon Mustard
1 heaped teaspoon

PREPARE THE BANGERS:

Place the almonds, pumpkin seeds, salt and pepper into the hand blender container and blitz for 20 seconds until it turns into a fine 'flour' (do not remove from the container). Scatter 1 level tablespoon of the 'flour' onto a large chopping board or clean work-surface. Remove the ends from the leek, peel the garlic and finely slice both. Dice the mushrooms into small pieces. Peel and remove the core from the apple and finely chop.

PREPARE THE GRAVY:

Peel the onion and slice thinly. Finely chop the thyme. Dissolve the stock in 200ml of boiling water.

PREPARE THE MASH:

Peel the potato, chop into small chunks and place in a pan.

MAKE THE GRAVY:

Heat the olive oil over a medium to high heat, add the onion and cook for 5 minutes. Add the stock, thyme, vinegar and mustard, reduce to a medium heat and simmer for 15 minutes with the lid off. Then reduce to a very low heat and continue to simmer until needed.

INGREDIENTS FOR THE 'GRAVY' AND 'THE MASH'
ON THE NEXT PAGE ≫•———➔

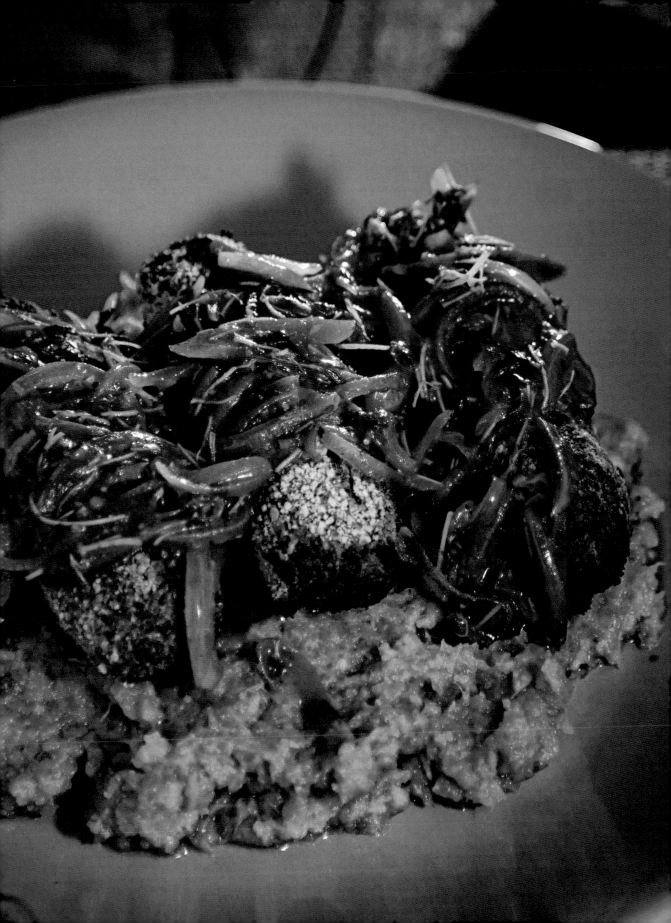

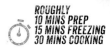

VEGGIE BANGERS 'N' MASH
WITH RED ONION GRAVY (CONTINUED)

GLUTEN-FREE

VEGAN

VEGETARIAN

CONTAINS NUTS

INGREDIENTS FOR THE GRAVY:

Red Onion
½ medium

Fresh Thyme
10g or 1 handful

Stock cube
1

Boiling Water
200ml/7fl oz

Olive Oil
1 tablespoon

Balsamic Vinegar
1 tablespoon

Dijon Mustard
½ teaspoon

INGREDIENTS FOR THE MASH:

Sweet Potato
3 medium

Boiling Water
1 litre/35fl oz

Olive Oil
½ tablespoon

Himalayan Rock Salt
1 pinch

Ground Black Pepper
1 generous pinch

MEANWHILE... MAKE THE MASH

Pour the boiling water over the potatoes, bring to the boil and cook for 15 minutes or until soft. Drain away the water, return the potatoes to the warm pan, add the oil, salt, pepper and mash. Replace the lid.

MEANWHILE... CREATE THE BANGERS:

Preheat the grill to a high heat.

Heat the oil in a frying pan over a medium to high heat. Add the leeks, garlic, mushrooms and apple and cook for 5 minutes stirring frequently. Then add the cooked ingredients to the 'flour' in the stick blender container along with the mustard and blitz for 10 seconds.

FREEZE:

Pop in the freezer for 15 minutes to firm.

CREATE:

Divide the mixture into 6 and using your (very clean!) hands, roll in to 6 fat sausages, then place on the pre-floured chopping board/work-surface and roll so they are lightly coated. Then place on a baking tray.

COOK:

Pop the baking tray under the grill and cook for 6-8 minutes, turning gently part way through.

SERVE:

Spoon the mash onto the plate, top with the sausages and finish with the lovely gravy.

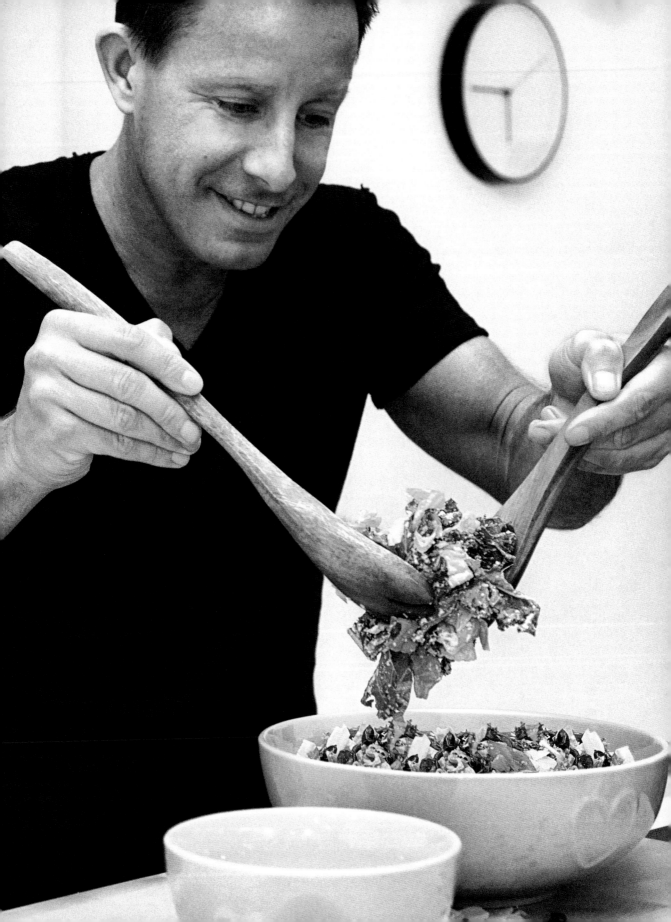

SUPER-PIMPED, SUPERFOOD CAESAR

The challenge was to take a classic such as the Caesar Salad that is traditionally fairly unhealthy compared to other salads and make it ultra nutritious. This salad is commonly made with fish (anchovies), dairy (parmesan and egg) and white bread (croutons) but I wanted to make it not only vegetarian, but also wheat and gluten free. I am very pleased to say that I think you will be suitably impressed! I've pimped it up, yet kept its essence and made it über healthy and utterly delicious. However, don't just take my word for it, try it for yourself...

GLUTEN-FREE

VEGETARIAN

CONTAINS NUTS

INGREDIENTS:

Serves 2

Pumpkin Seeds
30g or 1 handful

Himalayan Rock Salt
2 generous pinches

Curly Kale
50g or 1 large handful

Romaine Lettuce
1 small

Parmesan or Parmigiano Reggiano Cheese*
50g / 2oz

Cashew Nuts
60g or 1 large handful

Garlic
1 clove

Olive Oil
3 tablespoons

Dijon Mustard
1 flat teaspoon

Lemon (the juice of)
1

TOAST:

Heat a dry frying pan over a high heat and add the pumpkin seeds and 1 pinch of salt. Allow to toast for 1 – 2 minutes, shaking the pan frequently until the seeds start to brown, then remove from the heat.

PREPARE:

Remove the hard stems from the kale. Chop the lettuce into thick slices and remove the hard end. Shave the cheese using a vegetable peeler. Put the cashew nuts into a Super blend or hand blender and blend for a few seconds until the nuts turn to 'flour'. Peel the garlic and add to the mixing container along with the olive oil, mustard and lemon juice.

WHIZZ:

Blitz for 10 seconds until it forms a thick sauce.

CREATE:

Put the lettuce and kale into a mixing bowl, add the sauce and mix so all the leaves are coated. Then transfer to a salad bowl and sprinkle with the toasted pumpkin seeds and parmesan cheese.

* Leave out if Vegan
N.B Feel free to add some cooked salmon or chicken if you like.

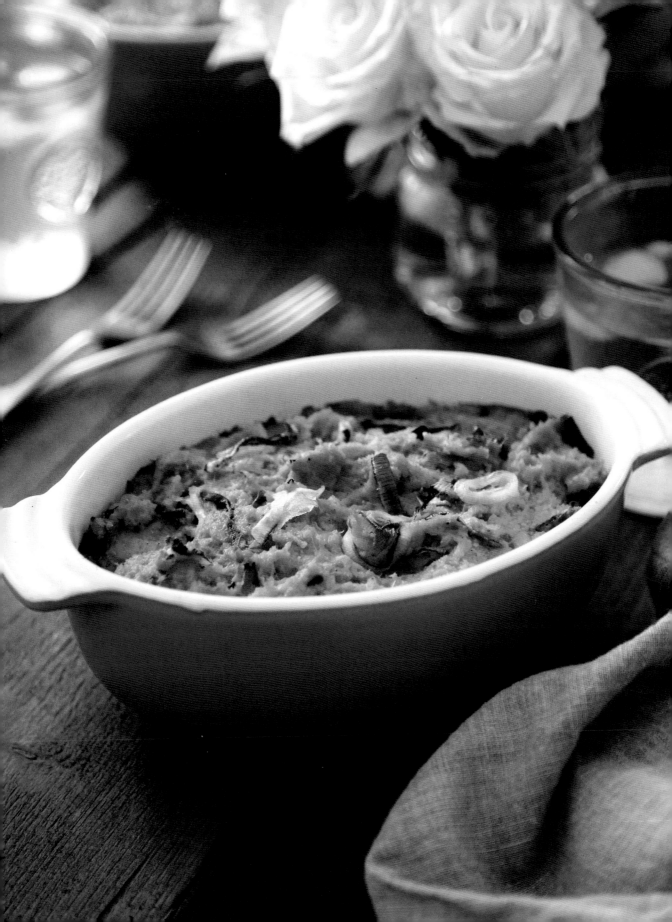

NO SHEEP SHEPHERD'S PIE!

If only Rachel from F.R.I.E.N.D.S had had this version to hand, she'd never have put mince in the trifle (sorry if you're not a F.R.I.E.N.D.S fan!) This is a true British classic, it's one of those extremely comforting dishes which immediately transports you back to childhood and makes you want to curl up on the sofa with a good book.

GLUTEN-FREE

VEGAN

VEGETARIAN

INGREDIENTS:

Serves 2

Red Onion
½ medium
Garlic
2 cloves
Sweet Potatoes
3 medium
Tomatoes
6 medium
Mushrooms
4 medium
Leek
1
Black Eyed Beans
120g/4oz or ½ tin
Olive Oil
2 tablespoons
Apple Cider Vinegar
1 tablespoon
Ground Cumin
1 teaspoon
Dijon Mustard
1 heaped teaspoon
Boiling Water
1 litre/35fl oz
Himalayan Rock Salt
1 pinch
Ground Black Pepper
1 generous pinch
Stock Cube
1

PREPARE:

Preheat the oven to 200 °C (400 °F/gas mark 6).

Remove the ends and skin from the onion, garlic and potato and dice the ingredients. Chop the tomatoes and mushrooms into small cubes. Remove the end from the leek and slice thinly. Drain and rinse the beans.

COOK:

Pour half the olive oil into a large pan and warm over a medium to high heat. Add the onion and garlic and cook for 5 minutes, stirring occasionally. Add the tomatoes, mushrooms, beans, vinegar, cumin and mustard, cover with a lid, reduce to a medium heat and cook for 15 minutes, stirring occasionally.

MEANWHILE...

Place the potatoes in a pan, cover with the boiling water and boil for 15 minutes until soft. Whilst the potatoes are cooking, heat the remaining olive oil in a frying pan and cook the leeks for 3 minutes or until they soften and start to brown.

MAKE THE MASH:

Once the potatoes are cooked, drain away the water, return the potatoes to the warm pan, add the salt and pepper and mash. Then add the cooked leek, gently combine and replace the lid.

THICKEN:

Once the vegetables have cooked for 15 minutes they will have released their juices, at this point, add the stock cube, stir well to ensure it is totally dissolved and continue to cook for a further 5 minutes with the lid off. Using a stick blender pulse for just 6 seconds, so that some of the sauce is blended to create a thicker sauce, but the majority is still in its original form. If you don't have a stick blender, you can blend 4 tablespoons in a regular blender and then return to the pan and mix well.

CREATE:

Pour the filling into an ovenproof dish, cover with the mash and leek topping and pop in the oven for 15 minutes to brown.

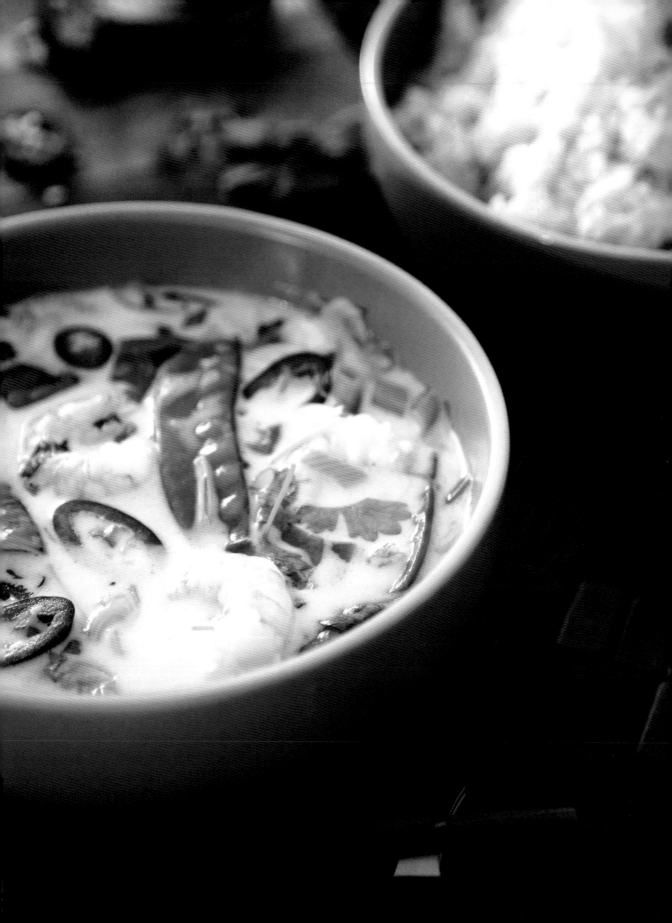

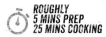
THAI GREEN PRAWN CURRY

GLUTEN-FREE

Up until the age of 40 I had consumed just three curries in my entire life. What put me off for years (and something I still don't understand), is the 'blow your head off' curries that are so hot, it's impossible to actually taste anything. This classic Thai Green Prawn Curry is perfectly balanced on the heat front. Yes, it has a kick, but it's calmed beautifully by the coconut milk and you can taste the full fusion of flavours that this wonderful dish has to offer. On the taste front it wins, but it's nutritionally where it stands out the most. It has 3 of the big guns of the superfood world; ginger, garlic and chilli. All 3 adding a 'Let Food Be Thy Medicine' element to this quick, easy and delicious curry.

INGREDIENTS:

Serves 2

Mange Tout
100g or 1 large handful
Garlic
2 cloves
Spring Onions
3 stems
Red Chilli
1 medium
Fresh Ginger
20g or 2 cm x 2 cm
Fresh Coriander
10g or 1 handful
Lemon Grass
1 stick
Basmati Rice
150g/5oz
Boiling Water
450ml/16fl oz
Coconut Oil
1 tablespoon
Coconut Milk
400ml/14fl oz or 1 can
Lime (the juice of)
1
Honey
1 teaspoon
Uncooked Prawns
200g/7oz
Himalayan Rock Salt
1 pinch

PREP:

Remove the ends from the mange tout. Remove the skin and hard end from the garlic and spring onion and slice thinly. Remove the top from the chilli and slice (keep the seeds in). Peel the ginger and finely slice. Coarsely chop the coriander. Remove the ends and outer layer of the lemongrass and bash with a rolling pin to release the flavours.
Rinse the rice.

BOIL:

Put the rice in a pan, add the water, bring to the boil, and cover with a lid, reduce the heat and simmer for 20 – 25 minutes, until the water has evaporated. Keep an eye on the rice and add a little more water if required.

MEANWHILE...

Heat the coconut oil over a medium to high heat and add the garlic, chilli and ginger. Cook for 2 minutes stirring occasionally. Add the coconut milk, lime, lemongrass and honey then reduce the heat, stir and simmer for 10 minutes. Add the mange tout and spring onions and cook for 2 minutes, then add half the coriander, prawns, salt and cook for 2 – 4 more minutes until the prawns turn pink and are therefore cooked.

SERVE:

Place the rice in a shallow bowl, add the curry and finish with the remaining coriander.

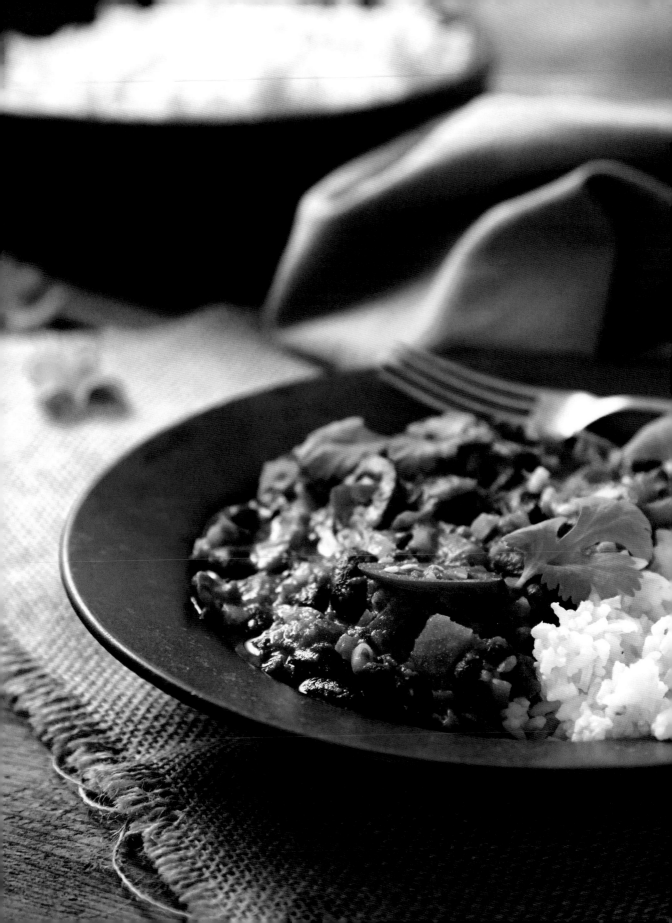

CHILLI-BEAN CHILLI

This chilli is hot, healthy and hearty. Beans themselves are so filling and 'meaty' in their own right, that even an avid meat eater might not notice the absence of the meat. I would recommend making a double batch of the chilli and popping half in the freezer ready for a cold winter evening.

GLUTEN-FREE

VEGAN

VEGETARIAN

INGREDIENTS:

Serves 2

Red Onion
½ medium

Garlic
2 cloves

Tomatoes
4 medium

Red Pepper
½ medium

Red Chilli
1 medium

Kidney Beans
240g/8.5oz or 1 tin

Basmati Rice
150g/5oz

Boiling Water
450ml/16fl oz

Olive Oil
1 tablespoon

Apple Cider Vinegar
1 tablespoon

Ground Cumin
1 pinch

Cayenne pepper
1 pinch

Dijon Mustard
1 heaped teaspoon

Honey*
2 teaspoons

PREPARE:

Remove the skin and hard ends from the onion and garlic and finely dice. Finely chop the tomatoes. Remove the core and seeds from the pepper and finely chop. Remove the top from the chilli and slice (do not remove the seeds). Drain the beans. Rinse the rice to remove the excess starch.

BOIL:

Put the rice in a pan, add the water, bring to the boil and cover with the lid. Reduce the heat and simmer for 20 – 25 minutes, until the water has evaporated. Keep an eye on the rice and add a little more water if required.

MEANWHILE...

Place the oil in a large pan and heat over a medium to high heat. Add the onion and garlic and cook for 5 minutes or until they soften. Add all other ingredients except the honey, reduce to a medium heat and allow to simmer for 20 minutes, stirring occasionally. Add the honey, then using a stick blender, pulse for just 6 seconds, so that some of the chilli is blended to create a thicker sauce, but the majority is still in its original form. If you don't have a stick blender, you can blend 4 tablespoons in a blender and then return to the pan and mix well.

SERVE:

Place a generous scoop of rice on your plate and pile the veggie chilli on top.

* If vegan just leave this out or use an alternative sweetener.

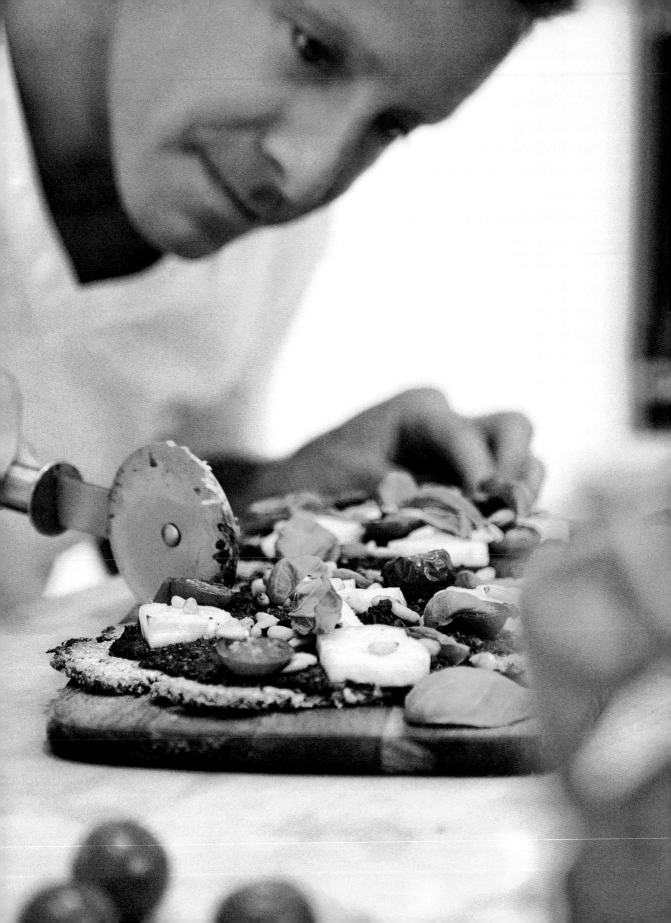

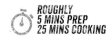

'NO DOUGH' HALLOUMI, BASIL & PINE NUT PIZZA

I have taken this Italian classic and removed all traces of dough (much to the horror of most Italians I am guessing!). My replacement dough is not just a substitute, it's an incredible alternative. If you think that it's impossible to make pizza without dough you are going to be pleasantly surprised. In fact I will go as far as to say once you make it, you'll be so impressed it will be one of those recipes you'll want to make for your friends time and time again.

GLUTEN-FREE

VEGETARIAN

CONTAINS NUTS

INGREDIENTS FOR THE BASE:

Serves 2 — 2 mini pizzas each

Parsnips
2 large
Oats*
120g/4oz
Cashew Nuts
100g or 2 handfuls
Himalayan Rock Salt
1 pinch
Black Pepper
1 pinch

SAUCE INGREDIENTS :

Garlic
2 cloves
Cherry Tomatoes
20
Fresh Basil
40g or 2 large handfuls
Sun-Dried Tomatoes
160g/6 oz
Balsamic Vinegar
2 tablespoons
Himalayan Rock Salt
1 pinch
Ground Black Pepper
1 generous pinch

TOPPING INGREDIENTS:

Halloumi
225g/8oz
Pine Nuts
20g/1oz

PREPARE:

Preheat the oven to 200 °C (400 °F/gas mark 6).
Line a large baking tray with greaseproof paper. Remove the ends and grate the parsnip.

IT'S ALL ABOUT THE BASE:

Place the oats, nuts, salt and pepper into the container of a Super Blend, hand blender or Bullet type blender and whiz for 10 seconds to form a 'flour'. Place the 'flour' into a mixing bowl along with the grated parsnip. Mix with your (clean) hands until the mixture turns into a dough. Divide the dough into four and flatten each one with your hands, then roll each one into a roundish shape using a rolling pin. Slide under each pizza base with a wide knife and transfer to the baking tray.

COOK:

Place the baking tray in the oven and cook for 15 minutes.

MEANWHILE...

Remove the ends and skin from the garlic and peel. Take 6 of the cherry tomatoes and cut in half. Remove the leaves from the basil and discard the stems. Slice the halloumi into small slices. Place the garlic, the whole cherry tomatoes, half the basil, the sun-dried tomatoes, vinegar, salt and pepper into the hand blender container, *Super Blend* or *Bullet blender* and blend for 10 seconds.

CREATE:

Spoon the sauce onto the cooked bases and spread evenly leaving a small gap around the edge. Randomly add the halloumi, the cut cherry tomatoes and pine nuts.

COOK:

Pop back in the oven for 10 minutes.

SERVE:

Remove from the oven and scatter with the remaining fresh basil.

*Oats are technically gluten-free but unfortunately some commercial oats have been cross contaminated with wheat, barley or rye, during the harvesting, storage, milling or processing, so be a little careful here if you are particularly sensitive.

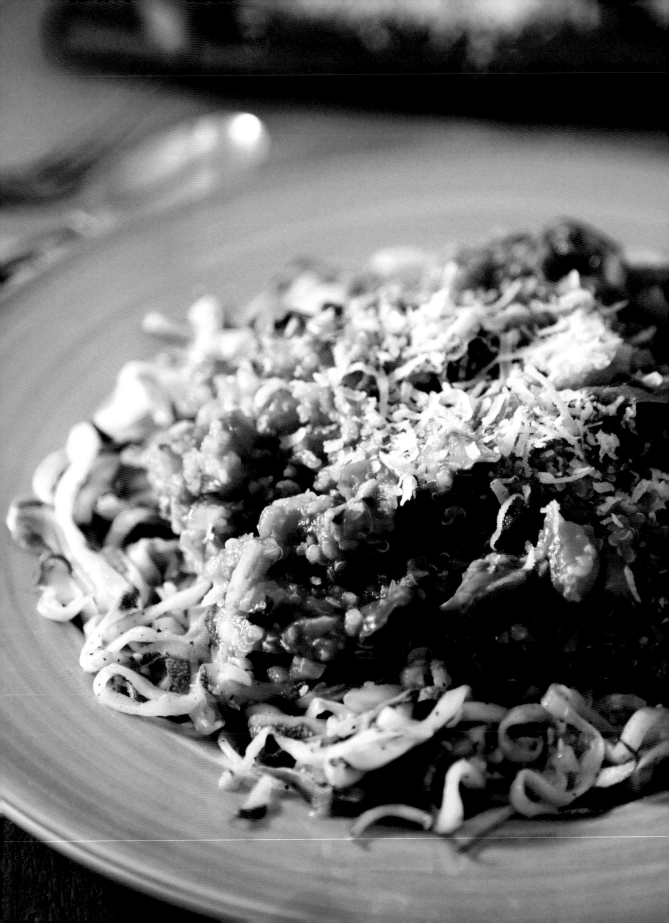

COURGETTI VEGGIE BOLOGNESE

The first time I had 'courgetti' was around 14 years ago at a David 'Avocado' Wolfe (he's a 'raw foodie' guy, who really knows his stuff!) seminar. It's like spaghetti, but made with courgettes using a little gadget called a spiralizer. It's surprisingly tasty and amazingly it tastes pretty close to actual spaghetti. It's gluten free by nature and, unlike most pasta, it won't leave you feeling bloated.

GLUTEN-FREE

VEGAN

VEGETARIAN

INGREDIENTS FOR THE 'PASTA':

Serves 2

Courgette/Zucchini
4 medium

Himalayan Rock Salt
2 generous pinches

Olive Oil
1 tablespoon

INGREDIENTS FOR THE BOLOGNESE:

Red Onion
½ medium

Garlic
2 cloves

Fresh Tomatoes
6 medium

Sun-Dried Tomatoes
150g/5oz

Red Pepper
1 medium

Fresh Basil
20g or 1 handful

Stock cube
1

Boiling Water
120ml/4fl oz

Olive Oil
1 tablespoon

Apple Cider Vinegar
1 tablespoon

Quinoa (or bulgur wheat/rice)
40g/1.5oz

Cayenne Pepper
1 pinch

Himalayan Rock Salt
1 generous pinch

Honey*
1 heaped teaspoon

Parmasean or Parmigiano Reggiano
Cheese (grated)**
50g/2oz

PREP THE 'PASTA':

Remove the hard end from the courgette and sprilize. Place the courgetti into a colander and pop on top of a mixing bowl. Sprinkle with the salt, mix and leave so that the salt draws out any excess water and tenderises the courgetti.

PREP FOR THE BOLOGNESE:

Remove the ends, peel and finely dice the onion and garlic. Finely chop the fresh and sun-dried tomatoes. Remove the core and seeds from the red pepper and finely chop. Roughly chop the basil, discarding any hard stems. Dissolve the stock cube in the boiling water.

MAKE THE BOLOGNESE:

Heat the oil over a medium to high heat, add the onion and garlic and cook for 5 minutes or until soft. Add the tomatoes, peppers, vinegar, quinoa, basil, cayenne pepper, salt and stock. Stir well, then reduce to a medium heat, cover with the lid and allow to simmer for 20 minutes, stirring occasionally. Finally add the honey and stir well.

MEANWHILE...

Pat the courgette dry with some kitchen roll to remove the excess moisture. Place the oil in a frying pan over a medium heat and add the courgetti. Cook for 2 – 3 minutes until warm, stirring constantly.

SERVE:

Place the courgetti onto the plate and add a generous spoonful of the veggie bolognaise and finish with a sprinkling of parmasean.

* If vegan use an alternative sweetener.
** Exclude if vegan.

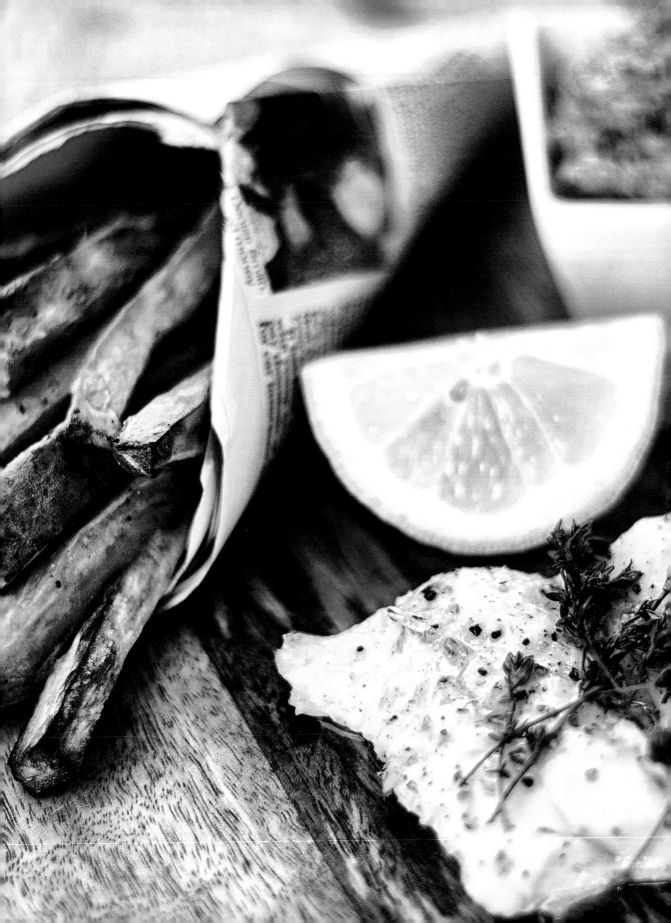

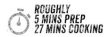
JASON'S CHEEKY FISH 'N' CHIPS WITH MINT PEA PUREE

GLUTEN-FREE

Yes indeedy there is a way to make a very healthy Fish 'n' Chips. This traditional Friday night British staple is usually deep fried and about as far away from 'health' as you can get. However, remove the batter, replace the white potatoes with the sweet variety, use the oven instead of a fryer and bingo – an unhealthy British classic made healthy. As this dish is a Friday night treat in the UK I have decided to stick with tradition and make this your Friday night, genuine treat. The addition of the Mint Pea Puree helps to lift this already amazing dish and is a far cry from the very 'mushy' and 'bland' peas served in your local chippy. It's Friday, without the fry!

INGREDIENTS:

Serves 2

Olive Oil
4 teaspoons

Himalayan Rock Salt
2 small pinches

Ground Black Pepper
2 generous pinches

Sweet Potato
2 large

Cod Fillet
2 x 150 – 200g / 5 – 7oz

Lemon
1.5

Fresh Thyme
1 large handful or 20g

Peas (fresh or frozen)
160g or 6oz

Fresh Mint
1 large handful or 20g

PREPARE:

Preheat the oven to 200 °C (400 °F / gas mark 6). Drizzle 2 teaspoon of olive oil onto a large baking tray, add a pinch of salt and pepper.
Cut the sweet potatoes lengthways into 'chips' (keep the skin on).

COOK:

Pop the baking tray in the oven for 2 minutes, remove, add the sweet potatoes, toss to ensure they are coated in oil, return to the oven and cook for 15 minutes.

MEANWHILE PREPARE:

Drizzle the remaining olive oil over both sides of the cod fillets, season with a pinch of salt and pepper and place skin down on a plate or board. Squeeze ½ a lemon over the cod and place the thyme on top. Remove the mint leaves from the stalks and discard the stalks.

COOK:

When the potatoes have cooked for 15 minutes, add the fish to the baking tray (skin side down) and cook for a further 10 minutes.

MEANWHILE...

Bring a pan of water to the boil and cook the peas for 3 – 4 minutes. Drain the peas and place in the container of a hand blender along with the mint leaves and juice from ½ a lemon. Blend until it forms a nice puree (if you feel you need a little more moisture, add a drop of water).

SERVE:

When the cod and sweet potatoes are cooked, remove from the oven, place on a plate and add the pea puree and squeeze the remaining fresh lemon over the fish.

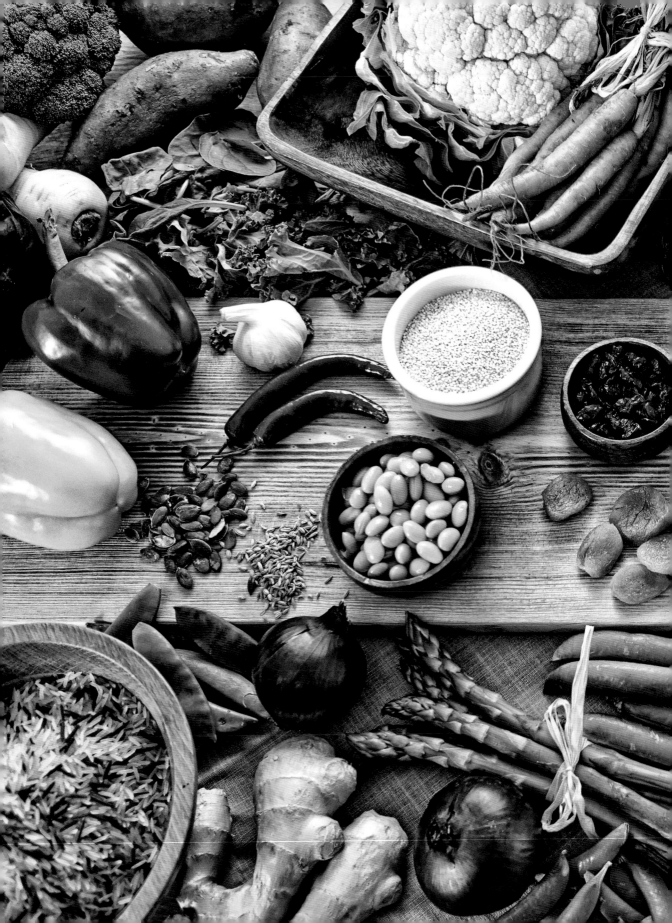

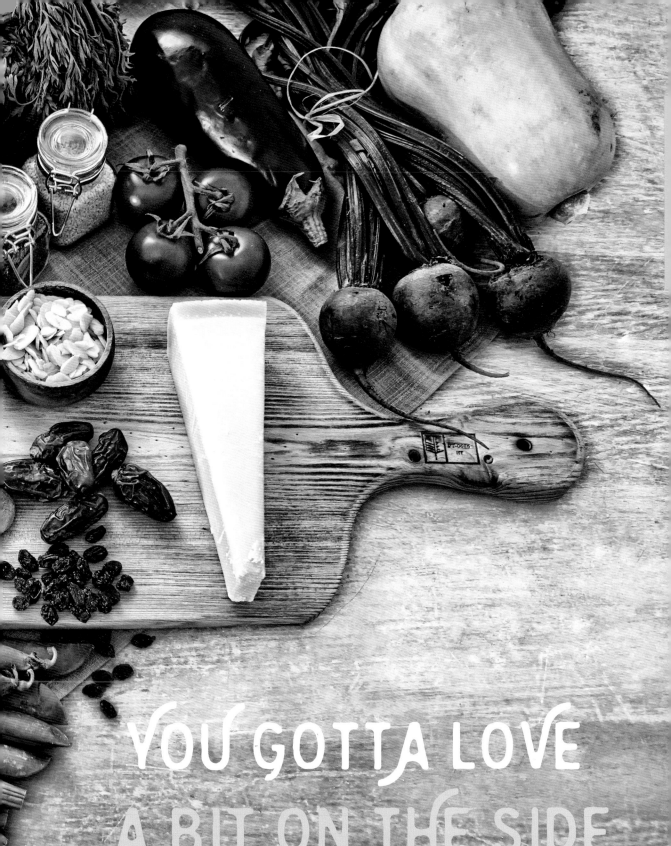

YOU GOTTA LOVE
A BIT ON THE SIDE

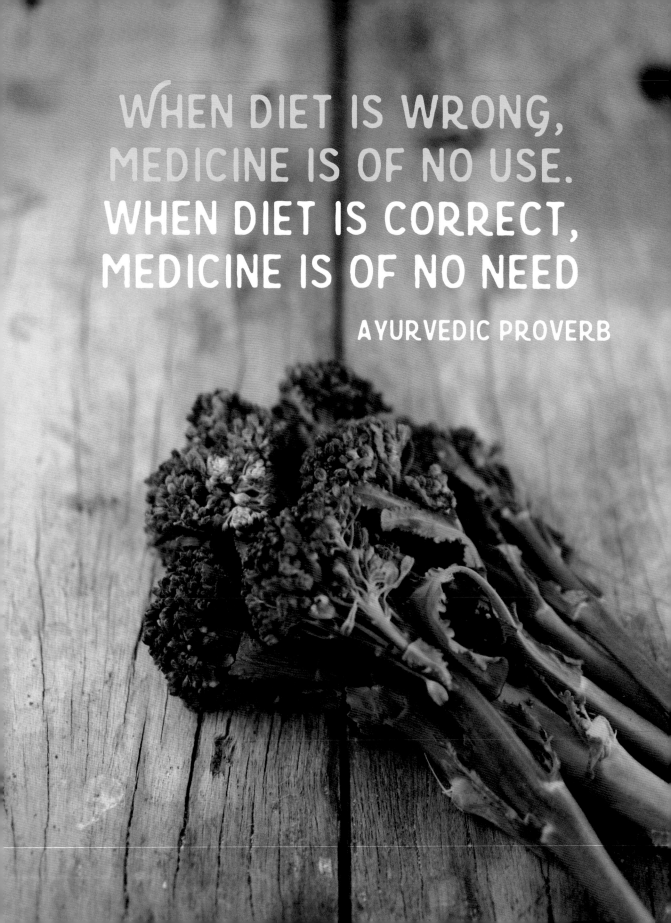

YOU GOTTA LOVE A BIT ON THE SIDE!

On a personal note, I love 'a bit on the side' (cue the *Carry On* music!) and many dishes just wouldn't hit the mark on either the filling, taste or nutritional front without them. Side dishes have saved me many times, whenever I couldn't find anything decent to eat on the mains section of a menu or when I wanted something a little naughty to accompany my healthy main course. One of the things I often do is have a main course salad and add some cheeky Sweet Chilli Potato Wedges (page 211) on the side. I get enough 'live' goodness from the big salad, so my nutritional needs are met, and I get my 'being human' needs met with the fries. Food isn't all about pure nutrition, it's also about being satisfied and for me anything slightly 'carby' hits that button!

Equally of course it works the other way around. It can often be the case where it's the main that's missing the 'live' goodness and 'a bit on the side' can really save the day on that front. Whilst all the recipes in this book are extremely healthy, clearly some are healthier than others. If you are having the Veggie Bangers 'N' Mash (page 185) for example, you may well want to do some Steamed Greens with Chilli & Fennel (page 209) as a side dish to add a little extra green goodness, or some Steamed Broccoli Spears with Soy Sauce & Sesame Seeds (page 223).

You'll also find:

* GRIDDLED ASPARAGUS WITH GINGER & PARMESAN (page 207)
* CHEESY VEGETABLE CHIPS (page 213)
* CARROT MASH WITH SALTED PUMPKIN SEEDS & BALSAMIC VINEGAR (page 219)

Then of course you have the option of turning some of the sides into starters or mains. This was something I used to do all the time when I first changed my eating habits and overnight went from a heavy meat eating, processed, take-a-way food junkie, to a complete vegan. When I went to restaurants I suddenly realised that most dishes were either meat, fish, loaded with dairy or heavily processed, so there was nothing for this new found vegan to eat. What rescued me was the sides menu and many a time I would ask for a few sides all on one large plate or I'd simply ask them to 'pimp my side' and turn one side dish into a main. I hope you enjoy a 'bit on the side' as much as I do!

Remember to snap a pic of whichever side you decide to make and share it on social media to spread the Super *fast* Food message and help to make a difference.

#superfastfood

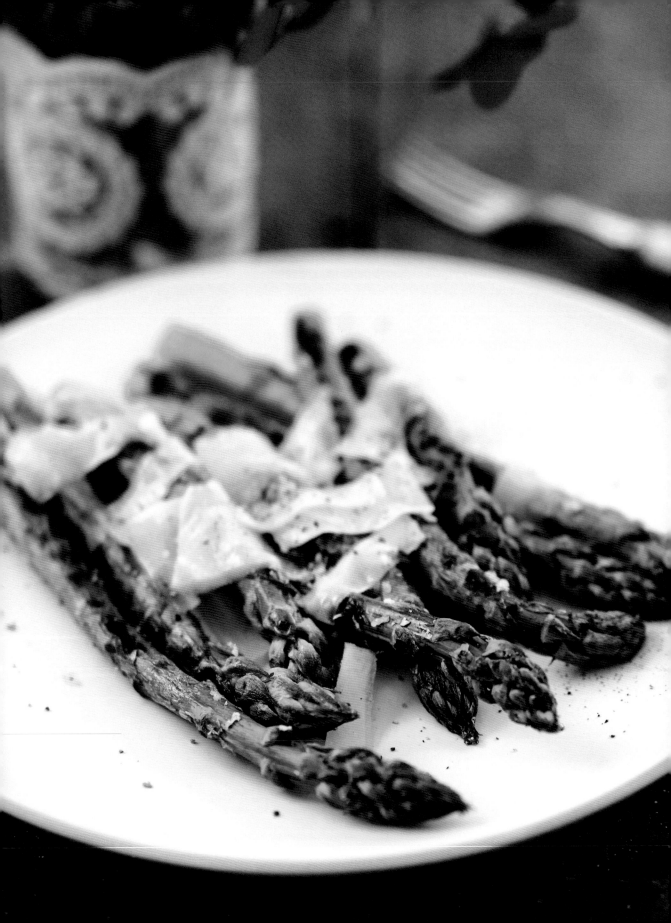

GLUTEN-FREE

VEGETARIAN

GRIDDLED ASPARAGUS WITH GINGER & PARMESAN

This wonderful 'bit on the side' is not just a pretty face. The asparagus is a very good source of fiber, folate, vitamins A, C, E and K, as well as chromium; a trace mineral that enhances the ability of insulin to transport glucose from the bloodstream into the cells. The ginger is known to have a positive effect on just about everything health related and parmesan adds that certain something to this wonderful side dish. I was a vegan for 4 years and I must say, grilled asparagus without the parmesan was like having fish and chips without the chips!

INGREDIENTS:

Serves 2

Asparagus
300g / 11oz

Fresh Ginger
30g or 2 cm x 4 cm

Parmesan or Parmigiano Reggiano Cheese
50g/2oz

Olive Oil
½ tablespoon

Ground Black Pepper
1 generous pinch

PREPARE:

Remove any hard ends from the asparagus. Peel the ginger and then grate using a small hand grater. Using a vegetable peeler, thinly slice the cheese.

GRIDDLE:

Place a griddle (or frying pan) over a high heat and when the pan is hot, add the asparagus, drizzle over the oil and allow to cook for 2 – 3 minutes. Then turn the asparagus, add the ginger and cook for a further 2 –3 minutes.

SERVE:

Remove from the pan and sprinkle with the cheese shavings and black pepper.

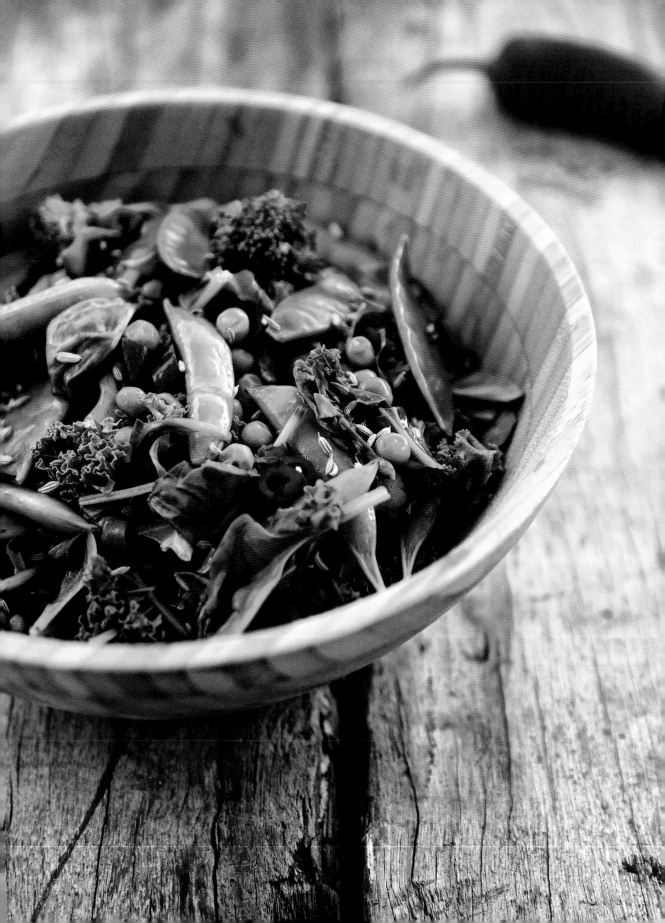

STEAMED GREENS WITH CHILLI & FENNEL

Nothing on earth would exist without the colour green, it is life essentially and we need a great deal of this colour food in our diets consistently. This is why it's a good idea to choose this as your 'bit on the side' more often than you do those spicy potato wedges or fries! The chilli and fennel really add something special to what could otherwise be accused of being a little bland. This is perhaps the most 'super side' of the bunch with the big players of the health world making a showing — broccoli, kale, spinach, mange tout and sugar snap peas; BOOM!

GLUTEN-FREE

VEGAN

VEGETARIAN

INGREDIENTS:

Serves 2

Chilli
1 medium

Mange Tout
60g or 1 small handful

Sugar Snap Peas
60g or 1 small handful

Broccoli
150g or 3 –4 florets

Kale
50g or 1 handful

Spinach
50g or 1 handful

Peas (fresh or frozen)
75g/3oz

Sesame Oil
1 tablespoon

Himalayan Rock Salt
1 pinch

Fennel Seeds
1 heaped teaspoon

PREPARE:

Remove the top from the chilli, cut in half and thinly slice (don't remove the seeds). Remove the ends and any stringy spines from the mange tout and sugar snap peas. Cut the broccoli florets into small bite sized pieces.

STEAM:

Place all the ingredients except the chilli, sesame oil, salt and fennel seeds into either an electric steamer or a pan steamer (you will need to add boiling water) and steam for 5 – 7 minutes, depending on your al dente preference.

SERVE:

Remove the veggies from the steamer, place in a serving bowl, add the sesame oil, chilli, salt and fennel seeds and mix well.

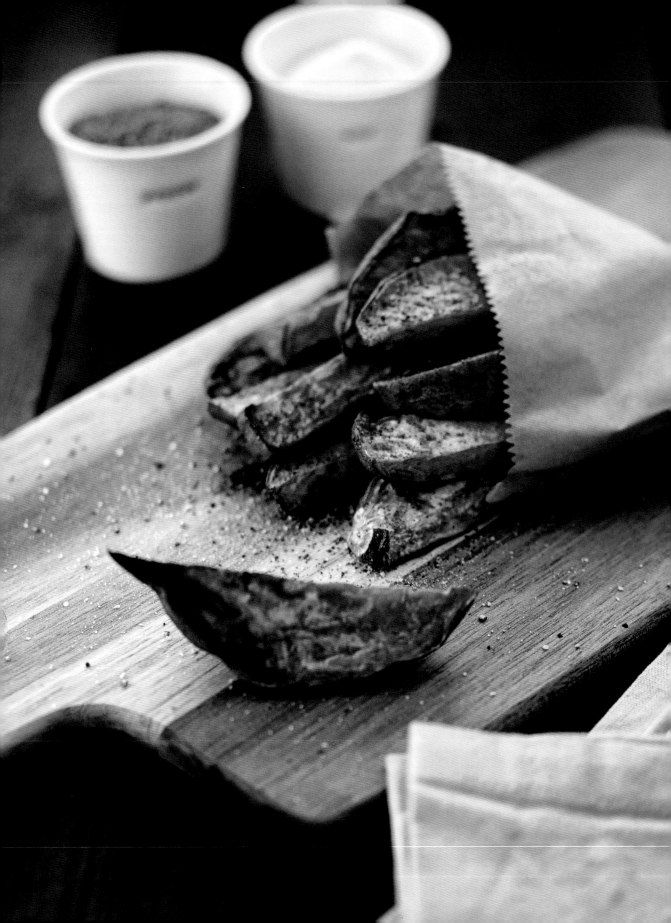

GLUTEN-FREE

VEGAN

VEGETARIAN

SWEET CHILLI POTATO WEDGES

In this book, I suggest adding these as a side...a lot. It's fair to say that wherever you see a salad, I pretty much make a suggestion that you are free to add a cheeky portion of these fiery babies. I love them, what can I say! They are so simple to make and a wonderful, healthier alternative to the standard white potato variety due to sweet potatoes not raising blood sugar as quickly. They are also perfect on their own when you're just chilling with a book or film — great with a little homemade pesto too!

INGREDIENTS:

Serves 2

Sweet Potatoes
2 large
Olive Oil
1 tablespoon
Cayenne Pepper
½ teaspoon

PREPARE:

Preheat the oven to 200 °C (400 °F/gas mark 6).

Cut the sweet potatoes into wedges and place in a mixing bowl. Add the olive oil and cayenne pepper and mix well. Place the coated potatoes onto a baking tray.

COOK:

Pop the baking tray in the oven and cook for 25 minutes.

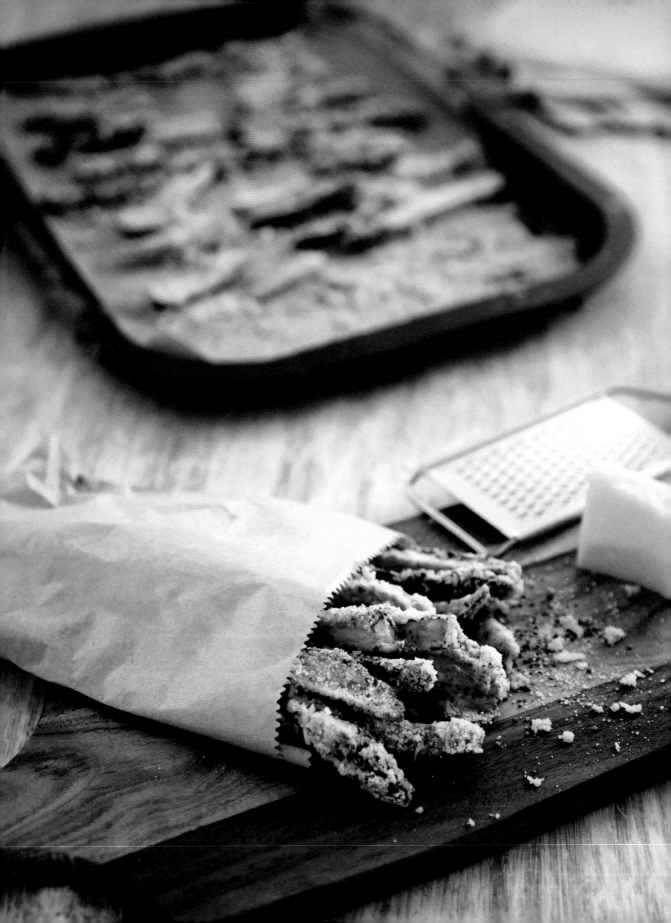

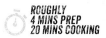

CHEESY VEGETABLE CHIPS

It's no secret; I love a hot chunky chip and if you ever see me in a restaurant, don't be surprised if you see a bowl of them on my table. The problem with this of course, is that hot white potato chips aren't exactly good for you! However, even though it's hard to get a healthy version when out and about, it couldn't be easier when you're at home. These go with, well — everything! Great as a side dish and ridiculously delicious when dipped into something like my homemade hummus.

GLUTEN-FREE

VEGETARIAN

CONTAINS NUTS

INGREDIENTS:

Serves 2

Sweet Potato
1 medium

Courgette / Zucchini
1 medium

Parsnip
1 medium

Asparagus
6 spears

Ground Almonds
60g / 2oz

Grated Parmesan or
Parmigiano Reggiano Cheese
40g / 1.5oz

Himalayan Rock Salt
2 pinches

Ground Black Pepper
3 generous pinches

Egg (Free-Range & Organic)
1 medium

PREPARE:

Preheat the oven to 200 °C (400 °F/gas mark 6).

Line a large baking tray with greaseproof paper.

Remove any hard ends from the vegetables and slice them all into thin chip size pieces (just cut the asparagus in half). Mix the almonds, cheese, salt and pepper in a large bowl. Whisk the egg. Dip the vegetable strips into the egg and then straight into the almond mix and place on the baking tray (not on top of each other).

COOK:

Put the baking tray in the oven and cook for 15 — 20 minutes until golden.

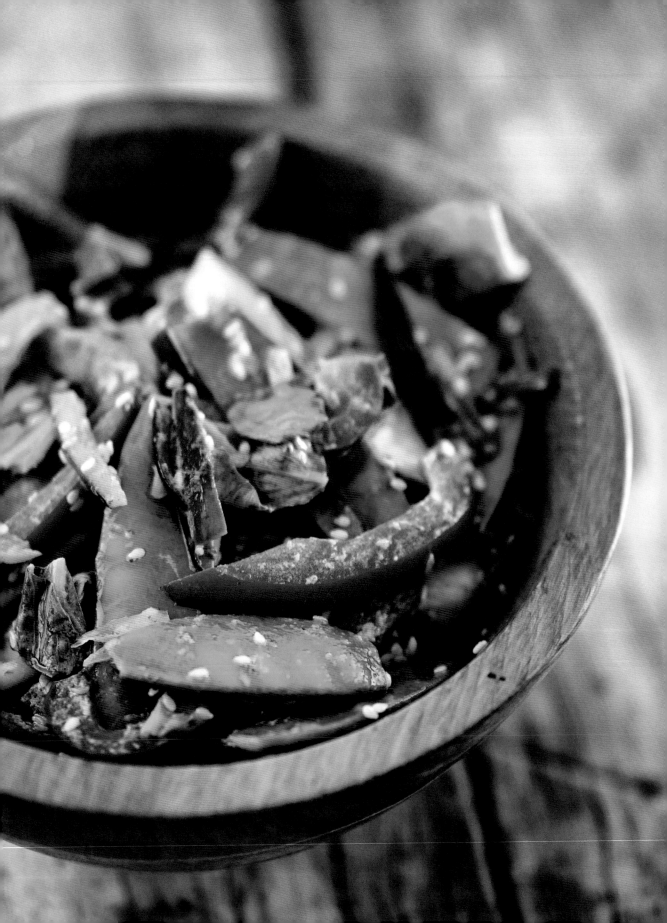

WOK FRIED VEG WITH SESAME, HONEY & TAHINI

GLUTEN FREE

VEGETARIAN

This 'bit on the side' would be equally at home as a main – all you'd need to do is double the ingredients and you'll have a seriously healthy meal. However, it's a truly wonderful side that compliments a lot of mains beautifully and takes a matter of minutes to make. Rich in vitamins, minerals, amino acids, essential fats, and good carbohydrates, it hits all of the right nutritional notes you'd expect from any recipe in this book.

INGREDIENTS:

Serves 2

Honey
1 heaped teaspoon

Tahini
1 heaped teaspoon

Red Onion
½ medium

Sugar Snap Peas or Mange Tout
40g or 1 small handful

Red Pepper
½ medium

Yellow Pepper
½ medium

Pak Choi
2 bulbs

Sesame Oil
1 tablespoon

Sesame Seeds
1 tablespoon

PREPARE:

Place the honey and tahini in a small bowl and mix.

Remove the ends and skin from the red onion, cut in half and slice thinly. Remove any hard ends and stringy spines from the mange tout or sugar snap peas. Remove the core and seeds from the peppers and thinly slice. Remove the ends from the pak choi and thinly slice.

COOK:

Put the oil in a wok (if you don't have one, you can use a frying pan) and place over a high heat. Add all the veggies except the pak choi and cook for 3 minutes, then add the pak choi and cook for a further 2 — 3 minutes (stirring frequently). Add the honey, tahini and sesame seeds, mix well and then remove from the heat.

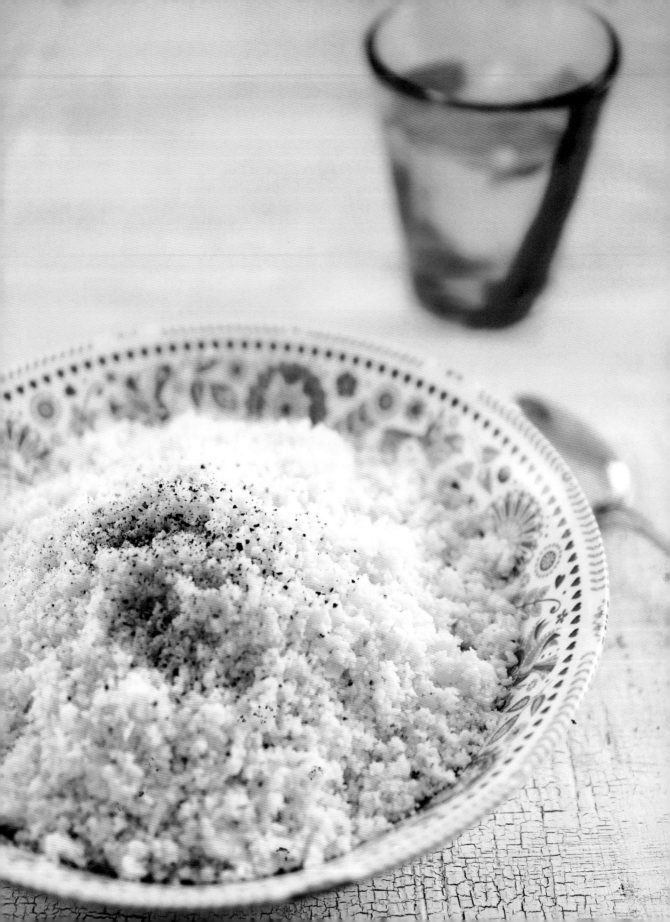

CAULIFLOWER 'RICE'

More and more people are becoming intolerant to grains. This is usually of the wheat variety, but many are also looking for an alternative to rice (often due to bleaching, processing and so on). We are looking to be more and more in control of everything we put into our body and cauliflower 'rice' is a great alternative to real rice and puts you fully in control of what's actually going in! This is stupidly easy to make and, unlike 'real' rice takes just 5 minutes to cook.

INGREDIENTS:

Serves 2

Cauliflower
1 medium
Olive Oil
1 tablespoon
Himalayan Rock Salt
1 pinch
Ground Black Pepper
1 generous pinch

PREPARE:

Remove the green leaves from the cauliflower and cut into quarters. Place in a food processor and pulse until all the cauliflower is broken down and resembles cooked rice. If you don't have a food processor you can do this in small batches using either a hand blender, *Retro Super Blend* or *Bullet* or you can grate the cauliflower using the large holes of a traditional grater.

HEAT:

Put the olive oil in a large frying pan over a medium heat and then add the cauliflower, salt and pepper and cook for 5 minutes, stirring frequently.

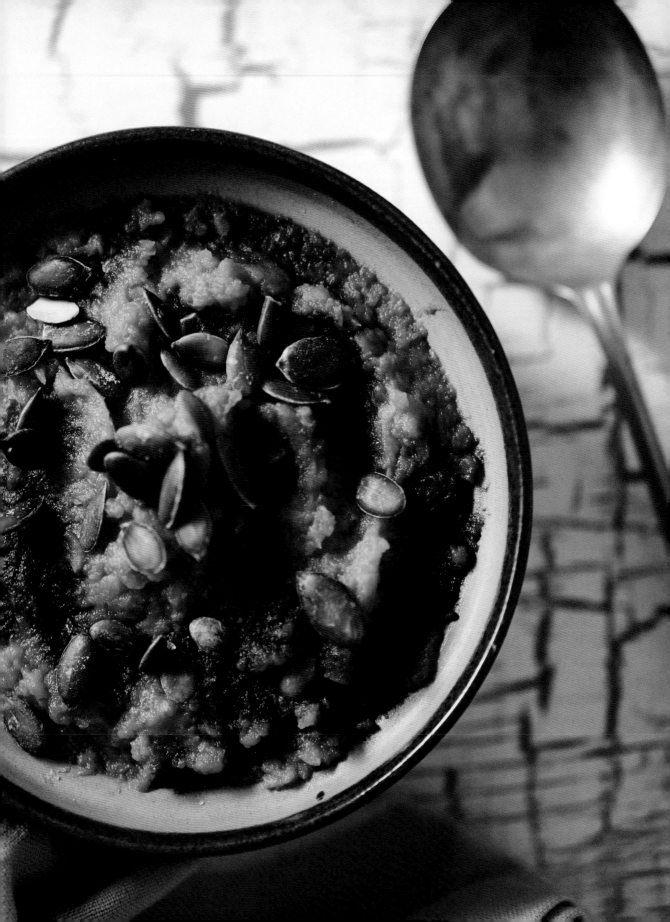

CARROT MASH WITH SALTED PUMPKIN SEEDS & BALSAMIC VINEGAR

GLUTEN-FREE

VEGAN

VEGETARIAN

Here we have a wonderful alternative to 'normal' white potato mash, which can often be extremely starchy and, well let's face it, fattening! The salted pumpkin seeds and balsamic vinegar add something quite unexpected, but in a very good way. No white potato, no butter, yet somehow it ends up with a creamy texture and tastes divine.

INGREDIENTS:

Serves 2

Carrots
6 large

Boiling Water
400ml/14fl oz

Pumpkin Seeds
1 tablespoon

Himalayan Rock Salt
1 generous pinch

Balsamic Vinegar
2 tablespoons

PREPARE:

Preheat the oven to 180 °C (gas mark 350 °F/gas mark 4).

Remove the ends and peel the carrots. Chop into small chunks, place in a pan and cover with the boiling water. Place the pumpkin seeds and salt on a baking tray.

COOK:

Cook the carrots over a medium to high heat for 10 minutes until soft. Place the pumpkin seeds in the oven for 5 minutes and then remove. When the carrots are cooked, remove from the heat, drain, return to the pan and pat with some kitchen roll to remove any excess water. Add half the balsamic vinegar and mash using a hand blender or food processor to make them lovely and smooth.

SERVE:

Place the carrot mash in a bowl, drizzle with the rest of the balsamic vinegar and sprinkle with the salted pumpkin seeds.

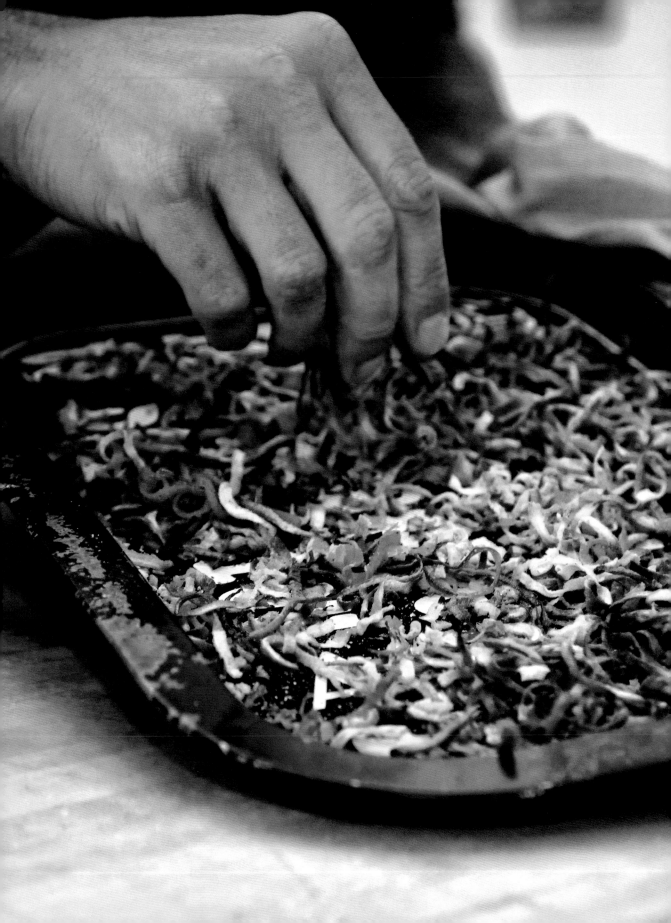

CURLY VEGGIE CRISPS

Be careful with these, yes they are good for you, but the saying of 'you can't have too much of a good thing' doesn't apply to food! These are incredibly delicious and extremely moreish, so be aware that however much you make, you'll most likely eat — especially whilst they're still hot. These are SO much better than regular crisps and, in my opinion, they taste better too. FYI, I have called these 'crisps' because I am still not ready to go completely to the U.S 'chips' side of life.

GLUTEN-FREE

VEGAN

VEGETARIAN

INGREDIENTS:

Serves 2

Sweet Potato
1 medium

Parsnip
1 medium

Carrot
1 medium

Olive Oil
2 tablespoons

Himalayan Rock Salt
2 generous pinches

Ground Pepper
2 generous pinches

PREPARE:

Preheat the oven to 200 °C (400 °F/gas mark 6).

Spiralize the vegetables. Place a large baking tray in the oven to warm. Put the olive oil and half of the salt into a mixing bowl, add the spiralized vegetables and toss until all are covered.

COOK:

Put the vegetables onto the baking tray, and cook for 20 minutes, turning 2 or 3 times to ensure they are crispy but not burnt!
Remove from the oven and sprinkle with the remaining salt and pepper.

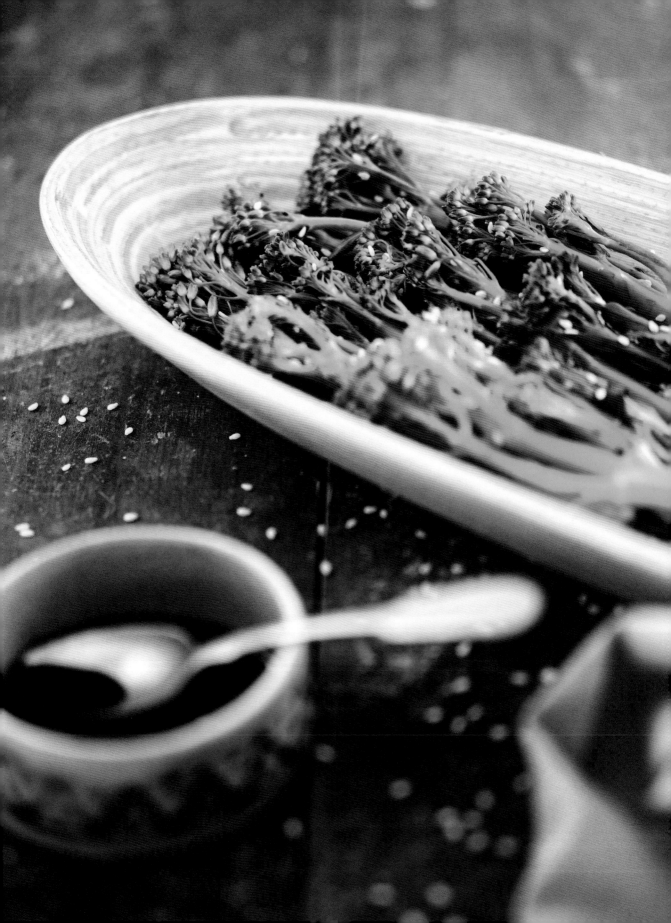

STEAMED BROCCOLI SPEARS WITH SOY SAUCE & SESAME SEEDS

VEGAN

VEGETARIAN

This is a side you'll come back to time and time again as, of all the superfoods on earth, broccoli will always remain near the top of the 'amazing for you' charts. In The Classics, I've got a Veggie Bangers 'n' Mash (page 185) and this side works beautifully with that, but then it works beautifully with many dishes — as you're about to discover.

INGREDIENTS:

Serves 2

Broccoli Spears
200g / 7oz
Boiling Water
400 ml / 14fl oz
Soy Sauce*
1 tablespoon
Sesame Seeds
1 tablespoon

PREPARE:

Place the broccoli and water in a steamer (pan or electric).

STEAM:

Steam for 5 — 7 minutes.

SERVE:

Remove the broccoli from the steamer, place in a serving bowl, drizzle with the soy sauce and sprinkle with the sesame seeds.

* If gluten free, use Tamari or Braggs Liquid Aminos.

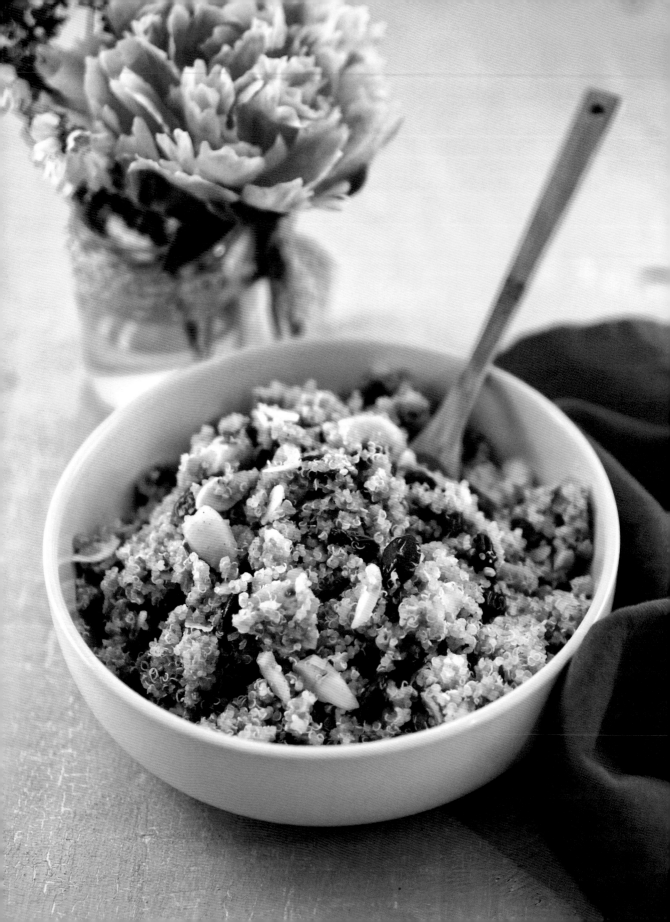

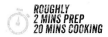

WARM FRUITY QUINOA

Quinoa is arguably the best alternative to wheat and perfect for anyone who happens to be gluten intolerant, (a number which is creeping up almost daily). This beautiful side tastes a little like the mini couscous salad you can get in M&S, but without the preservatives. The superfood fruits in this dish, transform an already good, but bland grain, into a power house of nutrition and taste. Quinoa is a complete protein as it contains all 9 essential amino acids required by the body.

GLUTEN-FREE

VEGAN

VEGETARIAN

CONTAINS NUTS

INGREDIENTS:

Serves 2

Dates (medjool are best)
6

Apricots (un-sulphured are best)
6

Quinoa
200g / 7oz

Cold Water
600ml / 21fl oz

Cranberries (dried)
25g or 1 small handful

Raisins
20g or 1 small handful

Almond Flakes
25g or 1 small handful

Ground Cinnamon
1 level teaspoon

Orange (the juice of)
1 medium

PREP:

Remove any hard ends and stones from the dates. Cut the dates and apricots into smallish pieces. Rinse the quinoa.

COOK:

Put the quinoa in a pan, add the water and bring to the boil, then reduce the heat and allow to simmer for 15 – 20 minutes. Be careful that the pan doesn't boil dry and if necessary add a little more water. At the end of the 20 minutes, if any water is remaining, simply drain away.

SERVE:

Add the dates, apricots, cranberries, raisins, almonds, cinnamon, orange juice and mix well. Enjoy whilst warm, or allow to cool.

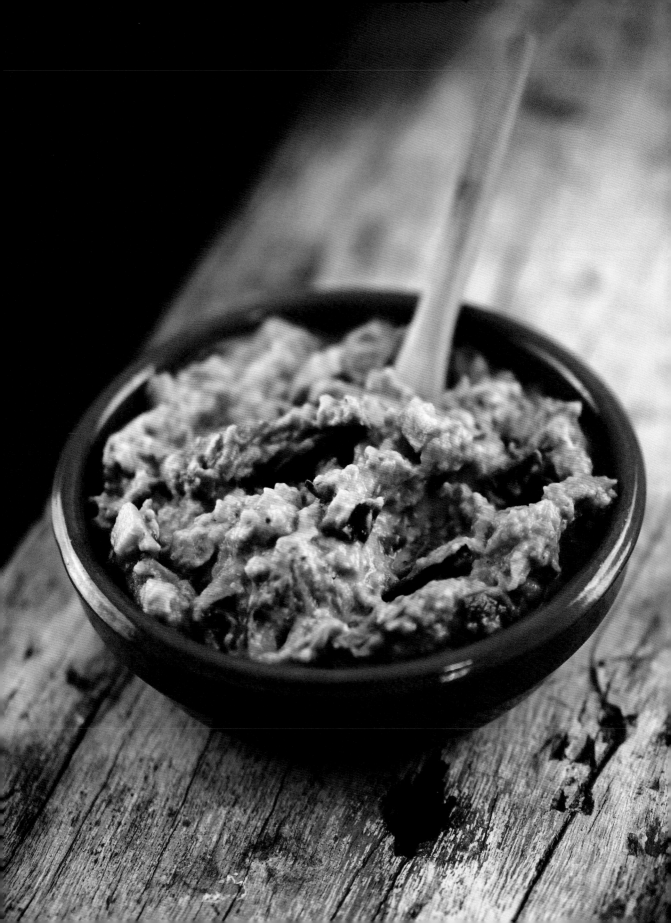

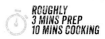

SPICY AUBERGINE WITH CREAMY GOATS CHEESE

GLUTEN-FREE

VEGETARIAN

Here's another dish which would be equally at home as a starter. It's a wicked side though and has the ability to really complement many a dish in this book. I'm slightly biased as I LOVE goats cheese!

INGREDIENTS:

Serves 2

Aubergine
1 medium

Tomatoes
2 medium

Goats Cheese (soft)
50g / 2oz

Coconut Oil
1 tablespoon

Cayenne Pepper
¾ teaspoon

PREPARE:

Remove the green top from the aubergine and then chop into small chunks along with the tomatoes and goats cheese.

COOK:

Put the coconut oil in a pan and place over a medium heat. Add the aubergine, tomatoes and cayenne pepper, stir and then cover with a lid and cook for 10 minutes, stirring frequently.

BLEND:

Add the goats cheese to the pan and using a stick blender pulse just enough to blend the goats cheese with the aubergine, whilst making sure to keep most of the aubergine and tomatoes whole (if you over blend, this will simply turn into a liquid!).

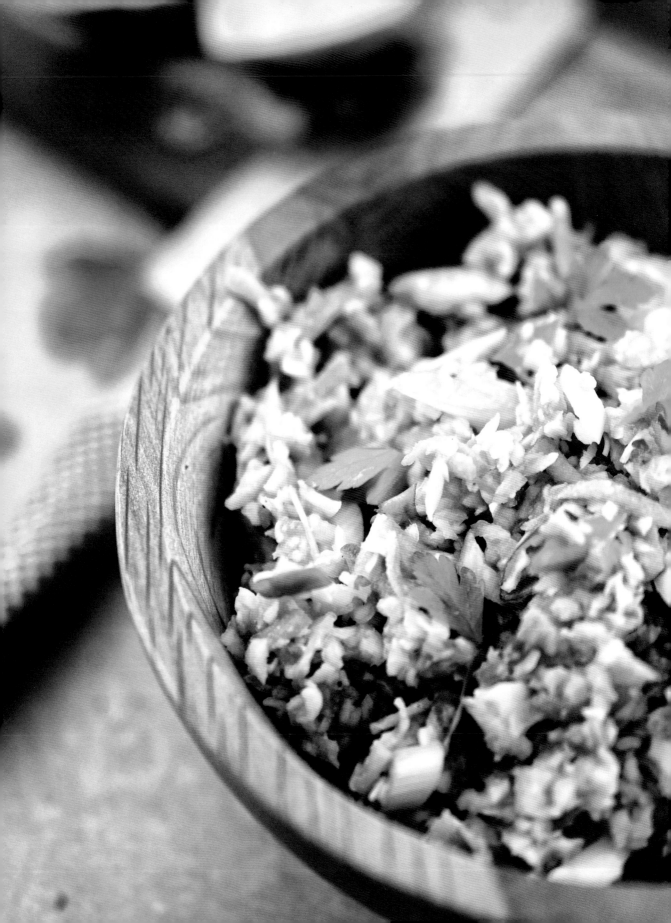

SUPER SLAW

Here's how to really raise the nutritional content of a classic 'bit on the side'. This has all the taste and texture of traditional coleslaw, but it's dairy-free and rich in essential fats, amino acids, vitamins and minerals. A genuine gorgeous take on the 'cole' original.

GLUTEN-FREE

VEGAN

VEGETARIAN

INGREDIENTS:

Serves 2

White Cabbage
¼ medium

Carrot
1 medium

Spring Onions
2 sprigs

Fresh Coriander
10g or 1 small handful

Himalayan Rock Salt
1 generous pinch

Ground Black Pepper
1 generous pinch

INGREDIENTS FOR THE DRESSING:

Avocado (ripe)
1 large

Limes (the juice of)
2

Dijon Mustard
1 heaped teaspoon

PREPARE:

Remove the core from the cabbage and the ends from the carrot. Grate the cabbage and carrot and place in a mixing bowl. Remove the end and outer skin from the spring onions and thinly slice. Roughly chop the coriander.

MAKE THE DRESSING:

Cut the avocado in half, scoop out the flesh (discard the stone) and place in a small mixing bowl. Add the lime juice, mustard and mash using a fork, don't worry if there are a few lumps and bumps in the sauce.

CREATE:

Combine all the ingredients in a large mixing bowl until all are coated.

SERVE:

This makes a great companion to any salad or the filling to a lovely roasted sweet potato.

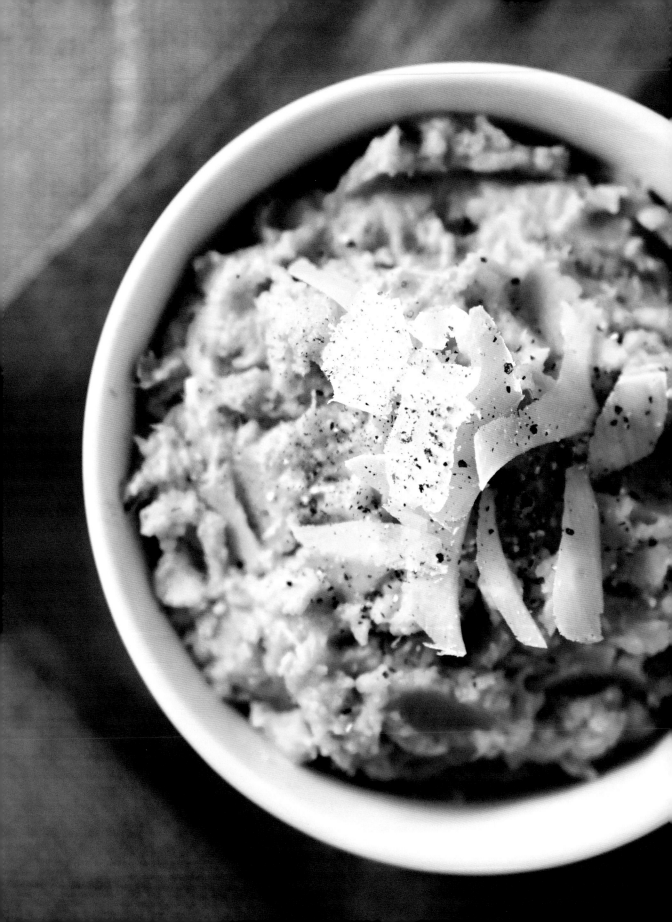

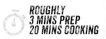

SWEET POTATO, GARLIC & PARMESAN MASH

So creamy, so delicious, so comforting, so good for you, so make some! You'll find I pair this up with a couple of mains in this book (such as 'Veggie Bangers 'n' Mash' page 185) but it can work with many dishes. The garlic adds the real superfood element, but the sweet potato is not to be sneezed at on the nutrient front either. This is one of those sides you'll come back to again and again for sure.

GLUTEN-FREE

VEGETARIAN

INGREDIENTS:

Serves 2

Garlic Cloves
4

Sweet Potatoes
2 medium

Parmesan or Parmigiano
Reggiano Cheese
50g/2oz

Boiling Water
1 litre/35fl oz

Ground Black Pepper
1 generous pinch

Himalayan Rock Salt
1 pinch

PREPARE:

Peel the garlic and the potatoes, removing any hard ends. Chop the potatoes into cubes and place in a pan with the garlic. Using a vegetable peeler, thinly slice the cheese.

BOIL:

Add the boiling water to the pan of potatoes and boil over a medium heat for 15 – 20 minutes, or until you can easily slide a knife into the potatoes. Remove the pan from the heat, drain away the water and pat dry with some kitchen roll.

SERVE:

Add the cheese, pepper and salt and mash thoroughly.

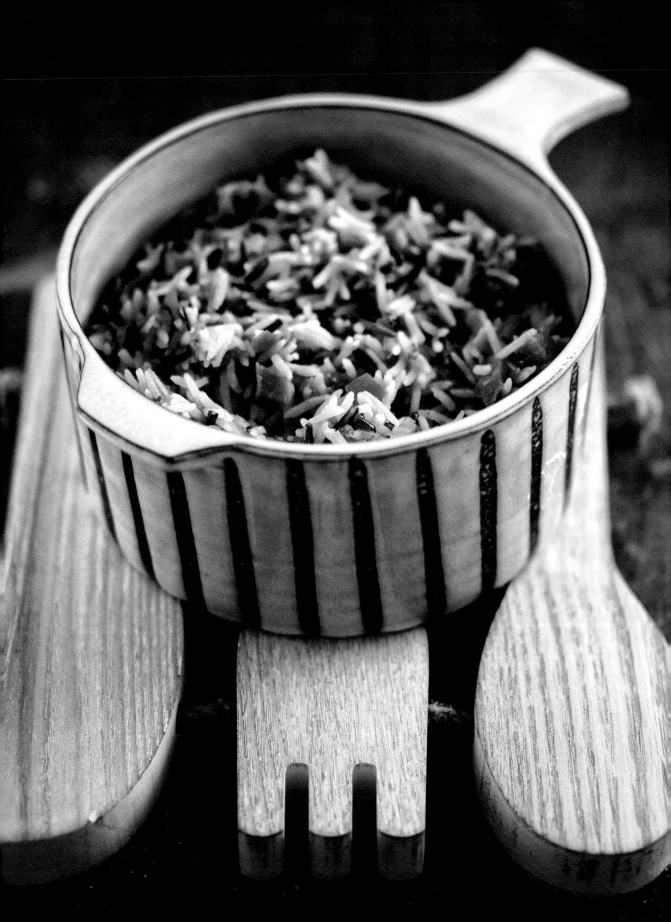

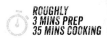

RICH TOMATO & WILD RICE INFUSION

This is more than just a little 'bit on the side' as you could easily make this as a main dish all on its own. I have teamed this up with my Pan Fried Chilli, Garlic and King Prawns (page 163) as it works a treat and clearly curry isn't really curry without a little rice. Wild rice is a staple in the East and once you add some garlic, onion, bell pepper and tomato, you lift it beautifully, not only on the taste front, but nutritionally you've just smashed it!

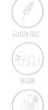

GLUTEN-FREE

VEGAN

VEGETARIAN

INGREDIENTS:

Serves 2

Red Onion
½ medium

Garlic
2 cloves

Red Pepper
½ medium

Tomatoes
4 medium

Wild Rice Combo*
150g / 5oz

Boiling Water
450m / 16oz

Sesame Oil
1 tablespoon

Apple Cider Vinegar
2 tablespoons

Honey**
½ tablespoon

Himalayan Rock Salt
1 large pinch

PREPARE:

Cut the ends off the red onion and garlic, peel and finely dice. Remove the seeds from the red pepper. Chop the pepper and tomatoes into small cubes. Rinse the rice, place in a pan and add the boiling water.

BOIL:

Bring the rice to the boil and then cover with a lid, reduce the heat and simmer for 20 – 25 minutes, until the water has evaporated. Keep an eye on the rice and add a little more water if required.

MEANWHILE...

Add the oil to a wok (or frying pan) and place over a medium to high heat. Add the garlic, red onion and red pepper and allow to cook for 10 minutes, stirring frequently. Then add the tomato and apple cider vinegar and cook for 20 minutes over a medium heat. Add the honey and salt, stir well and continue to cook for a further 5 minutes.

CREATE:

Drain away any remaining water from the rice, add to the tomato sauce and combine.

* Use a wild rice combo, such as wild rice & basmati, or wild rice & brown rice.
** If vegan either leave out or use alternative sweetener.

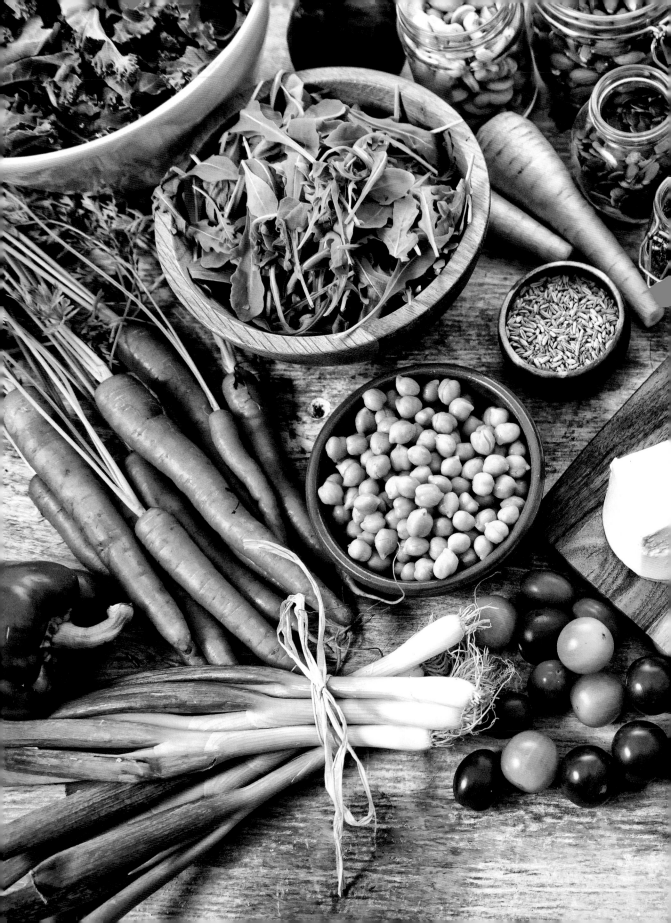

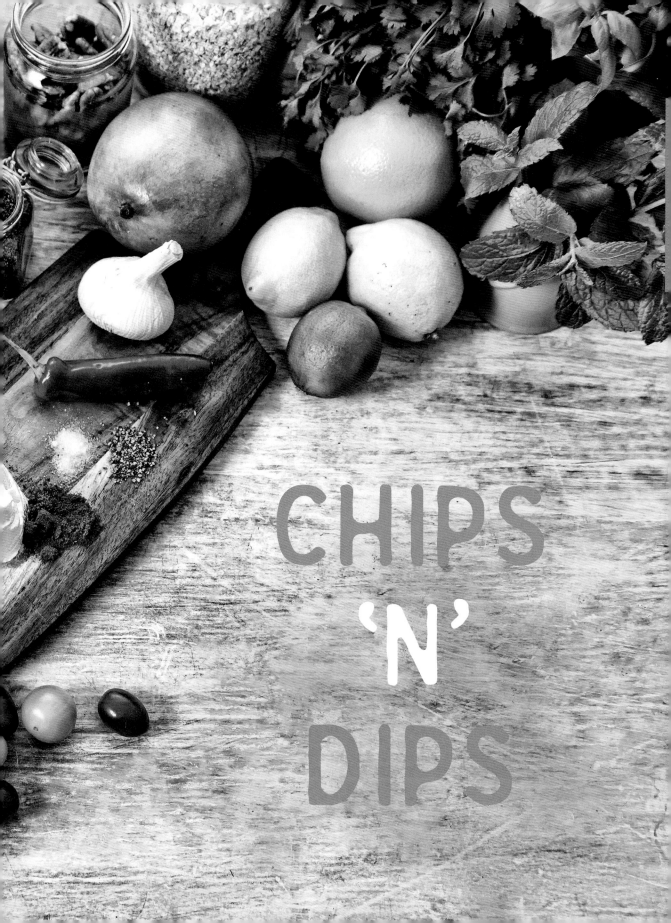

CHIPS 'N' DIPS

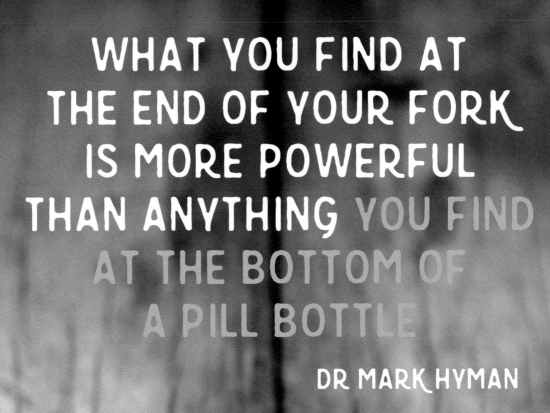
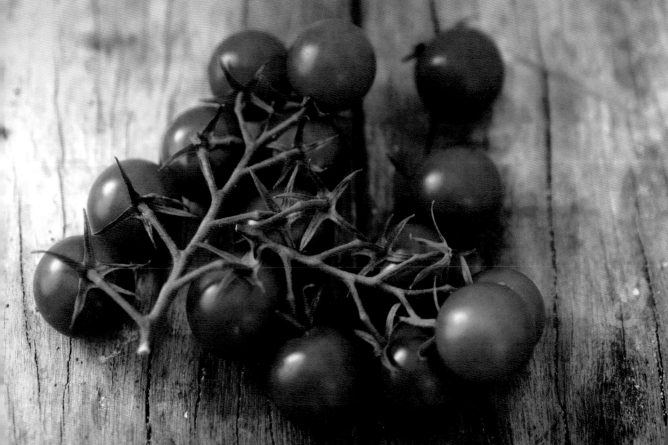

WHAT YOU FIND AT
THE END OF YOUR FORK
IS MORE POWERFUL
THAN ANYTHING YOU FIND
AT THE BOTTOM OF
A PILL BOTTLE

DR MARK HYMAN

ONCE YOU POP...YOU CAN STOP!

It's official, we are now so global and the world has shrunk to such an extent that the unthinkable has finally happened — 'crisps' are becoming 'chips'. Potato 'chips' are (or were) of course, a U.S of A 'thing' for what we call 'crisps' and what we call 'chips' they call 'fries' (although our 'fries' are much thicker and are, well, real British CHIPS!) To confuse the issue further (if I haven't already lost you at this point), in Australia they call them both 'chips'. Yes, they use the same name for potato 'chips' (or 'crisps') as they do for 'fries' (or 'chips'). They call 'fries' hot 'chips' and 'crisps' just 'chips'. It's all a bit of a head fry (see what I did there!) but it's clear we in the UK are caving in, with many of us now also referring to 'crisps' as 'chips' (I know, it's happening and I am as sorry as you are!) So to that end, and so people in the U.S and Aus don't get confused, I have called this section Chips 'n' Dips, even though clearly I am referring to 'crisps' and dips.

However, whatever you choose to call them, you can rest safe in the knowledge that all the 'chips 'n' dips' in this section are completely natural and chemical free. That cannot be said of some of the major players in the pre-packed potato 'chip' world, who even add MSG (Mono Sodium Glutamate) in a bid to make sure that 'once you pop', you won't be able to stop! Here you are in full control of the ingredients going in and you'll find that when your 'chips' and dips aren't loaded with chemicals (designed to make you want more and more), you can indeed stop once you've popped. This doesn't mean I've compromised on flavor and I would go as far as to say that this beautiful selection of natural 'chips 'n' dips' are far more flavorsome and delicious than their chemical covered cousins.

In this simple yet satisfying section you'll find:

The twists on hummus and salsa are to die for and the Goats Cheese & Basil Dip (page 243) you'll want to marry! All go beautifully with their 'dipping partners' of Natural Kale Chips (page 249). Nutty Seed Crackers (page 245) and Oat, Parsnip and Fennel Crackers (page 247). Enjoy!

Remember to snap a pic of you 'taking a dip' and share it on social media to help spread the Super *fast* Food message and help to make a difference.

#superfastfood

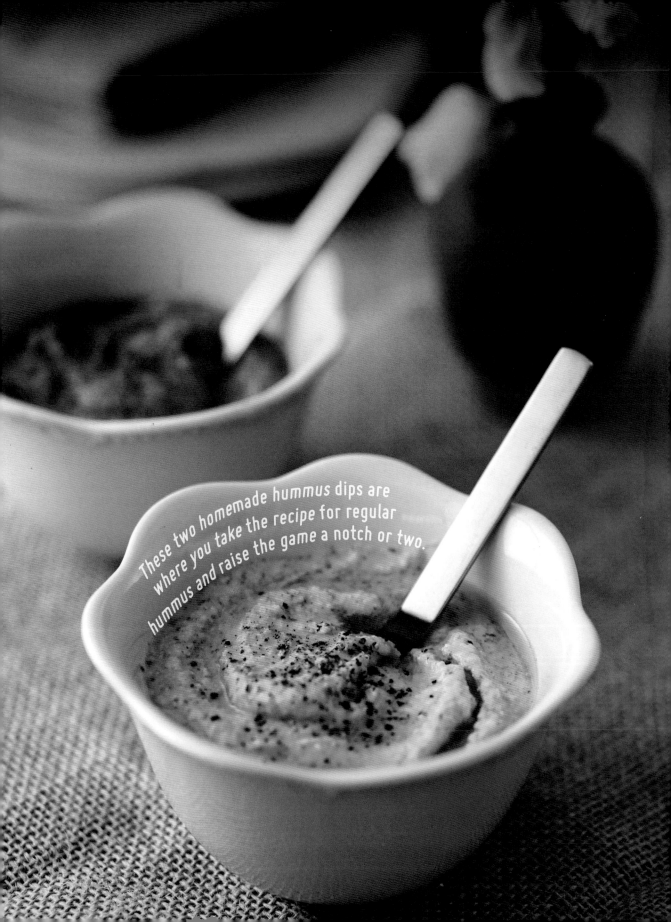

These two homemade hummus dips are where you take the recipe for regular hummus and raise the game a notch or two.

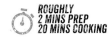

HUMMUS WITH A CHILLI & RED PEPPER KICK

INGREDIENTS:

Serves 2- 4

Red Chilli
1 medium

Red Pepper
1 medium

Olive Oil
100ml / 3.5 fl oz

Chickpeas
240g / 8.5oz or 1 tin (if using
uncooked, these will need
cooking first)

Lemon (the juice of)
1

Cayenne Pepper
1 pinch

Himalayan Rock Salt
1 small pinch

PREPARE:

Preheat the oven to 200 °C (400 °F/gas mark 6).

Cut the chilli and pepper in half and remove the top, core and seeds.
Chop the pepper into quarters and place in a baking tray along
with the chilli. Drizzle with a splash of the olive oil.

COOK:

Place the baking tray in the oven and cook for 20 minutes, turning the
peppers over, half way through.

BLITZ:

Drain the chickpeas and place in a *Super Blend* or the mixing container
of a hand blender. Add the cooked chilli, red pepper, remaining olive oil,
lemon juice, cayenne pepper and salt and blitz for about 60 seconds
until smooth.

SERVE:

Place into a dish and drizzle with a little olive oil.

GLUTEN-FREE

VEGAN

VEGETARIAN

MINT 'N' ROCKET HUMMUS

INGREDIENTS:

Serves 2 – 4

Butter Beans
235g/8oz or 1 tin

Fresh Mint (the leaves)
20g or 1 handful

Rocket.
80g or 2 large handfuls

Olive Oil
130ml/4.5fl oz

Himalayan Rock Salt
1 pinch

Ground Black Pepper
1 very generous pinch

COMBINE:

Drain and rinse the butter beans and place in a hand blender container
or food processor. Add all the other ingredients.

BLEND:

Blend for about 60 seconds until the hummus is lovely and creamy.

GLUTEN-FREE

VEGAN

VEGETARIAN

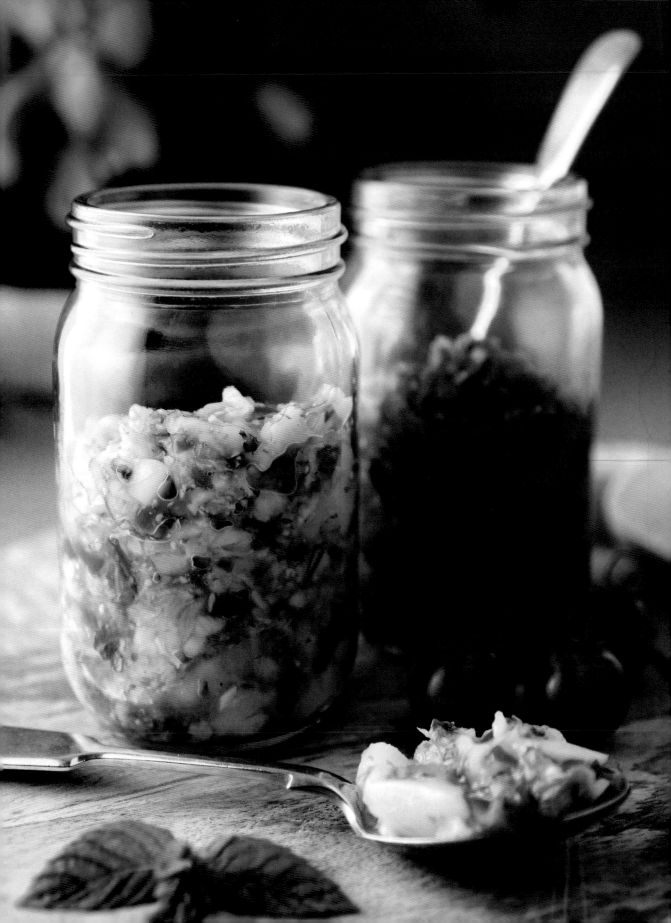

MANGO, ORANGE & CORIANDER SALSA

According to reports, more mangos are eaten fresh than any other fruit in the world and for good reason. Loaded with vitamins A, C and B, they have been shown to help lower cholesterol and have also been used as one of the natural weapons against many diseases, including the big C.

 GLUTEN-FREE

 VEGAN

 VEGETARIAN

INGREDIENTS:

Serves 2

Mango (ripe)
½

Orange
1 medium

Spring Onions
2 stalks

Cherry Tomatoes
8

Fresh Coriander
10g or 1 small handful

PREPARE:

Peel the mango, remove the flesh, discard the stone and cut into smallish pieces. Peel the orange, remove any hard fibres and seeds and chop into smallish chunks. Remove the ends and outer skin from the spring onions and slice thinly. Chop the cherry tomatoes into quarters.

PULSE:

Place all the ingredients in a mixing container of a hand blender or *Retro Super Blend* and pulse for just 4 pulses. Alternatively place all ingredients in a mixing bowl and mix vigorously for 1 – 2 minutes.

SIEVE:

Transfer the mixture to a sieve and allow any excess liquid to drain away. If you like, you can retain this liquid and add some water and ice to transform it into a nice cool drink. Meanwhile, the salsa is now ready to go.

TOMATO & RED PEPPER SALSA WITH A CHILLI KICK ROUGHLY 5 MINS

If you like a little fire in your dip, then this has it in abundance! 100% fresh and homemade, it's loaded with genuine 'live' nutrients and this combo is rich in vitamins. It will furnish the body with an array of goodness, whilst providing your taste buds with a touch of fiery warmth.

 GLUTEN-FREE

 VEGAN

VEGETARIAN

INGREDIENTS:

Serves 2

Red Onion
½ medium

Red Pepper
½ medium

Red Chilli
1 medium

Cherry Tomatoes
8 (red and also orange or yellow if possible)

Fresh Mint
20g or 1 handful

Lime (the juice of)
1

Himalayan Rock Salt
1 Pinch

PREPARE:

Remove the ends and skin from the red onion and finely dice. Remove the core and seeds from the red pepper and chop into small pieces. Cut the red chilli in half; remove the top and seeds and finely dice. Chop the cherry tomatoes into quarters. Remove the leaves from the mint (discard the stems) and roughly chop.

PULSE:

Place all the ingredients in a mixing container of a hand blender or *Retro Super Blend* and pulse for just 6 pulses. Alternatively, place all ingredients in a mixing bowl and mix vigorously for 1 – 2 minutes.

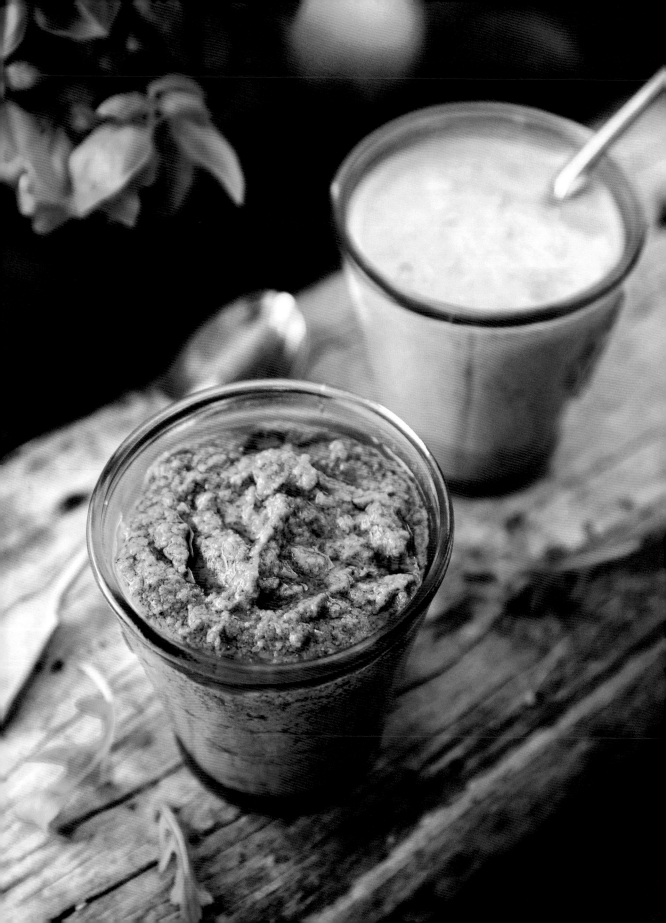

GOATS CHEESE & BASIL DIP

GLUTEN-FREE

VEGETARIAN

As I have already mentioned in some of the recipes throughout this book, I'm a little partial to goats cheese, so it won't come as a surprise that there's a dip that contains this beautiful, creamy and tangy cheese. The fresh basil, lemon juice, black pepper and salt all combine to make this one of my favourite dips of all time! All of these fresh ingredients contain a variety of vitamins and minerals, with calcium taking the limelight on this occasion. **Perfect with my** Nutty Seeded Crackers **found on** page 245

INGREDIENTS:

Serves 2

Fresh Basil
50g or 1 large handful
Goats Cheese (soft type, preferably with no skin)
125g/4.5oz
Olive Oil
1 tablespoon
Lemon (the juice of)
½
Black Pepper
1 generous pinch
Himalayan Rock Salt
1 pinch

PREPARE:

Remove any hard stems from the basil.

WHIZ:

Place all the ingredients in the container of a hand blender or *Retro Super Blend* and whiz for 20 – 30 seconds until all is combined.

SERVE:

Scoop into a nice little bowl and enjoy with some crackers — page 245

CREAMY, ZESTY ROCKET PESTO

GLUTEN-FREE

VEGAN

VEGETARIAN

CONTAINS NUTS

Pesto is an extremely versatile 'dip' or 'sauce'. It's the perfect partner for pasta, yet is equally at home as a little dip with chips. You can make pesto with all kinds of herbs; here I have used wonderfully nutritious rocket and added some cashew nuts. Cashews add an extra creaminess as well as amino acids and essential fatty acids. The touch of lime juice adds that wonderful citrus bite which makes all the difference. Rocket is loaded with folates as well as vitamins A, C and K.

INGREDIENTS:

Serves 2

Cashew Nuts
80g or 2 handfuls
Lime (the juice of)
1
Rocket
50g or 1 large handful
Olive Oil
100ml/3.5fl oz
Himalayan Rock Salt
1 pinch
Ground Black Pepper
1 generous pinch

BLEND:

Place the nuts in the container of a hand blender or *Bullet / Retro Super Blend* and whizz for 10 seconds until the nuts are ground. Add the other ingredients and whizz for a further 30 seconds until smooth.

SERVE:

Scoop into a bowl and enjoy with some sliced cucumber or crackers – page 245

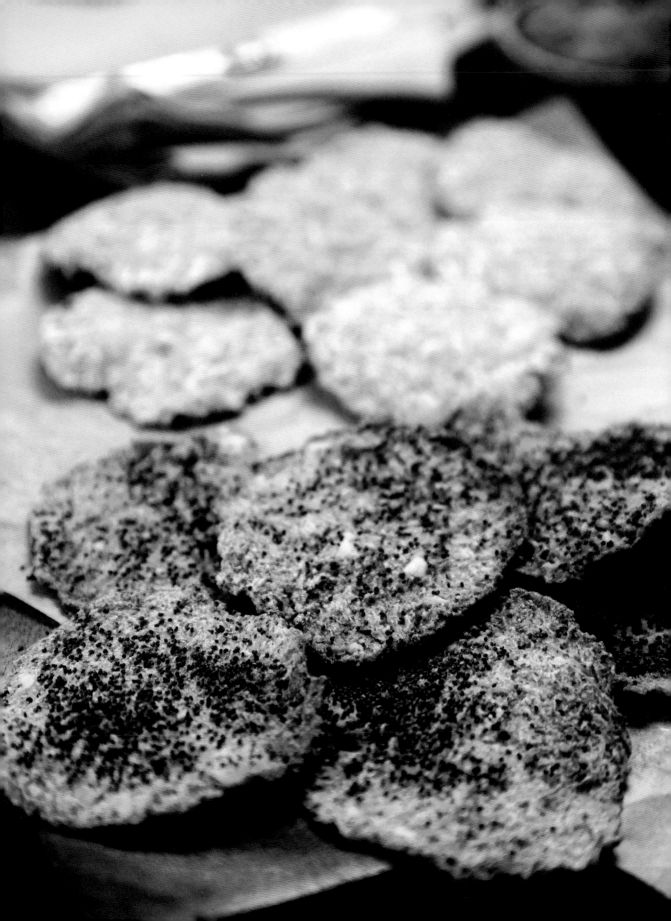

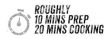

NUTTY SEEDED CRACKERS

Most people have never made their own dipping crackers and once you do, you'll be hooked. They're easy to make, taste delicious and are loaded with good nutrition — especially 'good' fats and amino acids (the building blocks for protein). These essential fatty acids are, as the name suggests, essential and are particularly good for the skin. This is a great protein and 'good fat' cracker that tastes delicious with any dip, especially homemade hummus.

GLUTEN-FREE

VEGAN

VEGETARIAN

CONTAINS NUTS

INGREDIENTS:

Makes 8 — 12 crackers

Carrots
1 medium
Almonds
30g or 1 small handful
Cashews
30g or 1 small handful
Pumpkin Seeds
25g or 1 small handful
Himalayan Rock Salt
1 pinch
Black Pepper
4 pinches
Poppy Seeds
½ teaspoon

PREPARE:

Preheat the oven to 160 °C (320 °F/gas mark 3).
Line a baking tray with greaseproof paper.
Remove the ends from the carrot and then grate using a wide grater.

BLEND:

Place the almonds, cashews, pumpkin seeds, salt and pepper into the container of a hand blender or *Bullet / Retro Super Blend* and whiz for 10 seconds. Place all the ingredients (except the poppy seeds) in a bowl and mix using a wooden spoon, then continue combining using your (clean!) hands, until it forms a dough-like consistency (add a small dash of water if needed).

CREATE:

Take a teaspoon of the mixture at a time, roll into balls and place on the baking tray; cover all the balls with a second sheet of greaseproof paper and press down on each ball so it flattens to the thickness of a cracker. Then remove the top sheet of paper and sprinkle with the poppy seeds.

COOK:

Place in the oven for 15 — 20 minutes until cooked, (timings will vary depending on the thickness).

SERVE:

Allow to completely cool and then peel the greaseproof paper away from each cracker. Enjoy with any of the dips on pages 239-249.

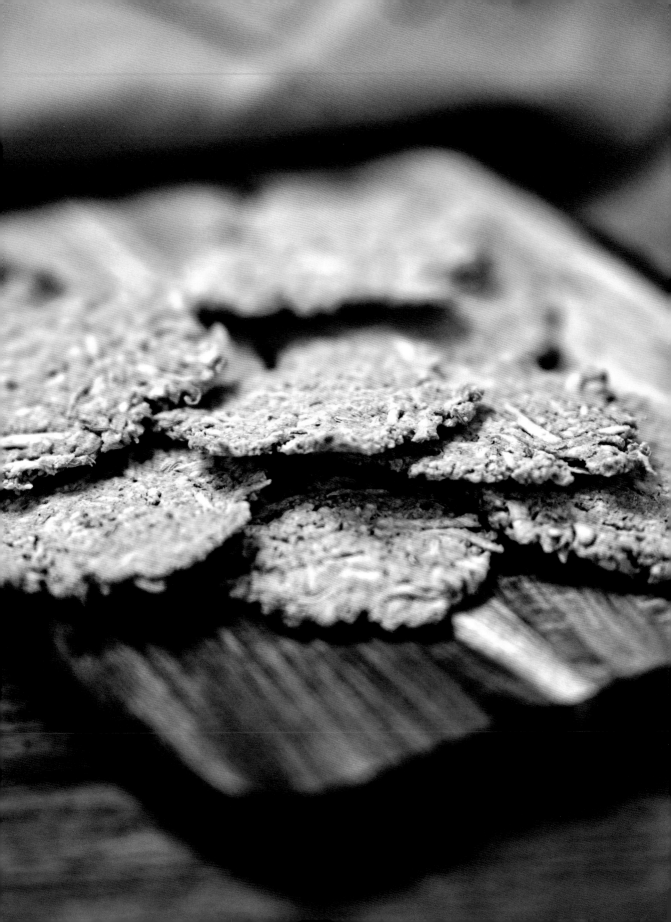

OAT, PARSNIP AND FENNEL CRACKERS

These are SO nice! Rich in vitamin A, essential fats and amino acids, these light yet filling crackers go stunningly well with the Goats Cheese and Basil Dip. You can also simply spread some nice ripe avocado over them; add a little lemon juice and some black pepper and boom, you've just produced one of the healthiest snacks around.

GLUTEN-FREE

VEGAN

VEGETARIAN

CONTAINS NUTS

INGREDIENTS:

Makes 8 — 12 crackers

Parsnip
1 medium
Oats*
50g/2oz
Cashews
30g or 1 small handful
Fennel Seeds
2 teaspoons
Himalayan Rock Salt
1 pinch
Black Pepper
1 pinch

PREPARE:

Preheat the oven to 160 °C (320 °F/gas mark 4).
Line a baking tray with greaseproof paper.
Remove the ends of the parsnip and grate using a wide grater.

BLITZ:

Place the oats, cashews, fennel seeds, salt and pepper into the container of a hand blender or *Retro Super Blend / Bullet* and whiz for 10 seconds. Place all the ingredients in a mixing bowl and mix with a wooden spoon and then your (clean!) hands for 1 — 3 minutes until it forms a dough (add a small dash of water if needed).

CREATE:

Take a teaspoon of the mixture, roll it into a ball and place on the baking tray (repeat with the rest of the mixture until it's all used up), cover with another sheet of greaseproof paper, press down on the balls so they flatten into crackers, then remove the top sheet of paper.

COOK:

Place in the oven for 25 - 30 minutes till firm, (cooking times will vary depending on how thick the crackers are).

SERVE:

Allow to fully cool before peeling off the greaseproof paper, enjoy with any of the dips on pages 239-249.

*Oats are technically gluten-free but unfortunately some commercial oats have been cross contaminated with wheat, barley or rye, during the harvesting, storage, milling or processing, so be a little careful here if you are particularly sensitive.

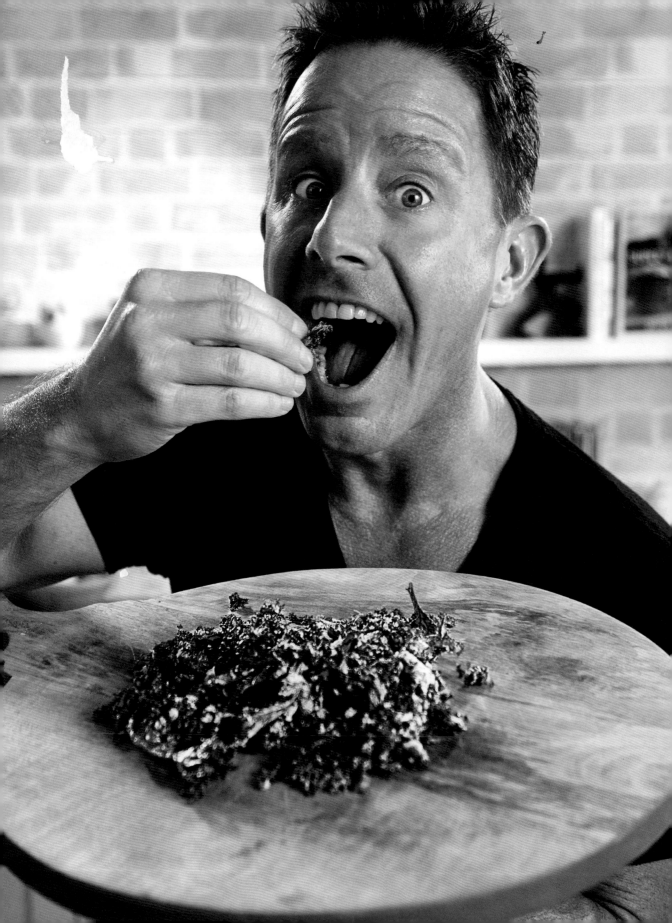

'HAIL THE KALE' CHIPS WITH A CREAMY CHILLI TOP

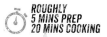

GLUTEN-FREE

VEGAN

VEGETARIAN

I once did one of those cheesy American infomercials and during the 'show', after making a beautiful juice with kale in, I had to raise a glass with one of the guests and literally say 'hail the kale'. I look back and question how and why I was ever persuaded to do such a thing, but it has at least inspired the name of these gorgeous 'chips' (aka crisps). Kale is in itself a powerful superfood but it doesn't even come close to the power of the garlic and chilli in this dip. These two ingredients leave most other superfoods in their wake. This recipe is actually quite clever as it's a 'chip' and a dip all combined!

INGREDIENTS:

Serves 2

Curly Kale
120g or 2 large handfuls
Chilli
1 medium
Garlic
2 cloves
Cashew Nuts
80g or 2 handfuls
Olive Oil
3 tablespoons
Lemon (the juice of)
2
Himalayan Rock Salt
1 generous pinch

PREPARE:

Preheat the oven to 140 °C (280 °F/gas mark 1).

Remove any hard stalks from the kale, place in a mixing bowl and put to one side. Remove the top of the chilli, cut into quarters and remove the seeds. Peel the garlic, remove any hard ends and cut into small chunks.

GRIND:

Put the nuts into a mixing container of a hand blender or *Bullet / Super Blend* and whizz for 10 seconds until the nuts are ground. Add the remaining ingredients (except the kale) and whizz for 20 — 30 seconds until smooth.

COMBINE:

Add the mixture to the kale and mix well (with your lovely clean hands) so all ingredients are combined.

COOK:

Spread the coated kale over a large baking tray and bake for 20 minutes, turning half way through.

ENJOY:

These kale chips are delicious served either straight out of the oven or cold.

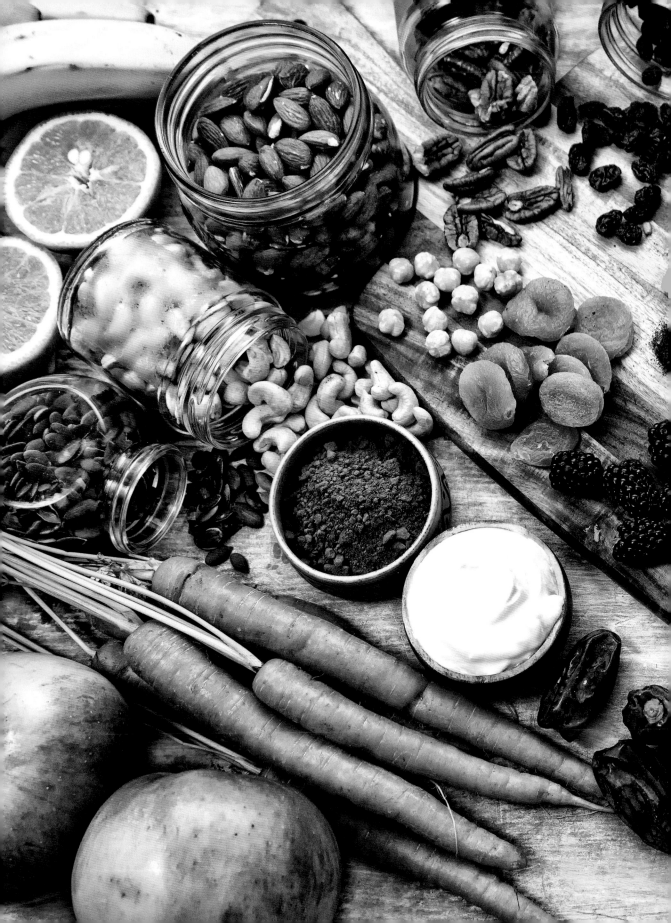

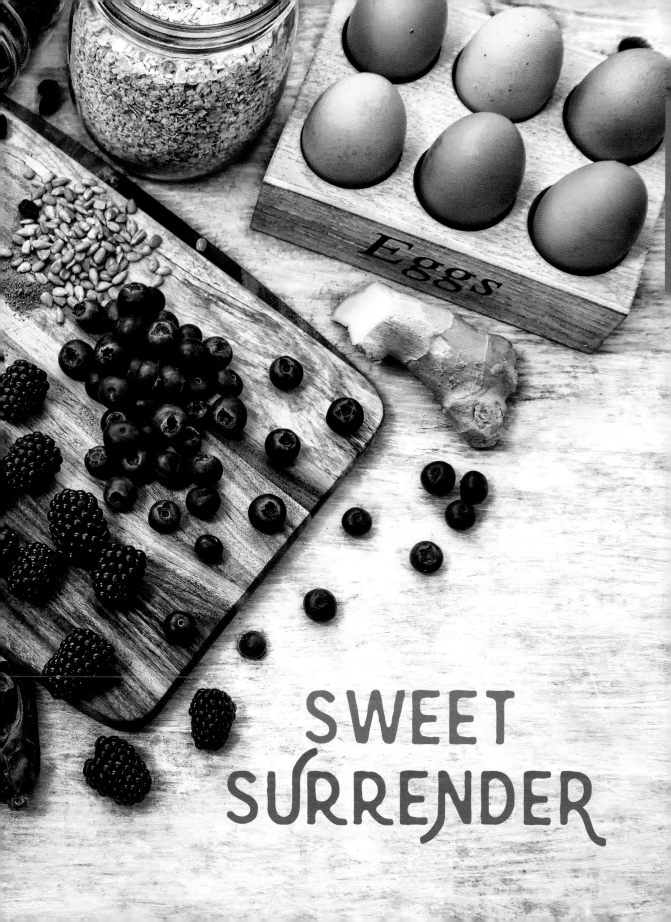

SWEET
SURRENDER

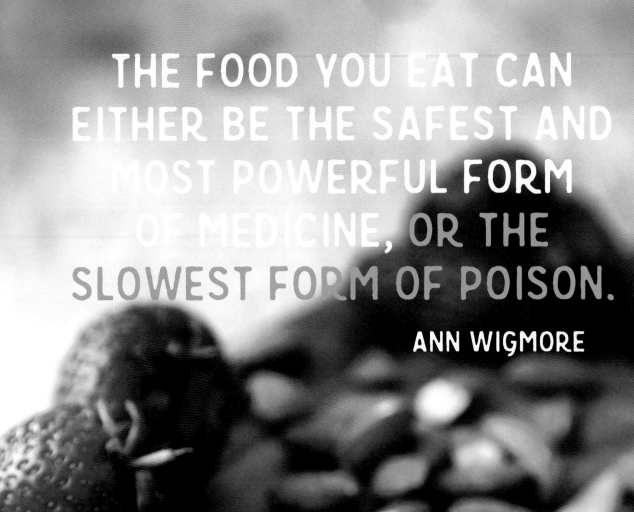

THE FOOD YOU EAT CAN EITHER BE THE SAFEST AND MOST POWERFUL FORM OF MEDICINE, OR THE SLOWEST FORM OF POISON.

ANN WIGMORE

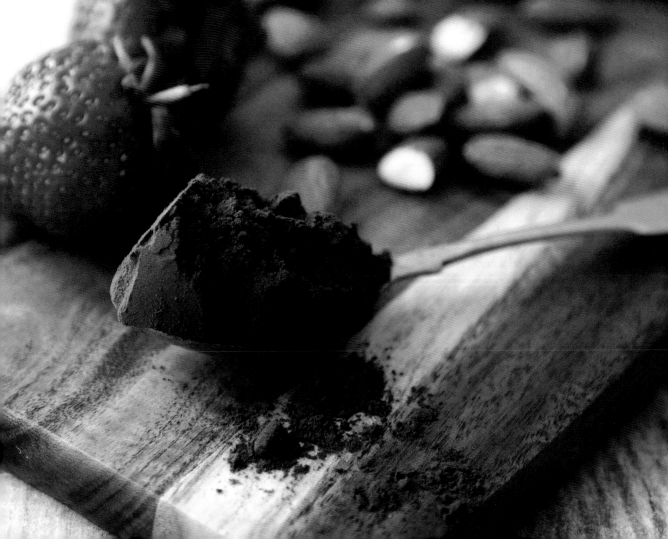

A LITTLE OF WHAT YOU FANCY!

If you have a sweet tooth and want life to consist of more than just salad and quinoa, then you've definitely come to the right section. We've all heard the saying, **'A little of what you fancy does you good'** and in this section you'll certainly find plenty of what you fancy, all of which are full of the 'good stuff'. I was always of the belief that if it tastes ridiculously good, it can't be doing you good, until of course I made some of these babies! Even though they are all full of goodness, please still take note of the 'little' in 'a 'little of what you fancy does you good' as it is indeed possible to have 'too much of a good thing', even when using natural ingredients. Dates are high in natural sugar and almond butter can raise the calorie bar up a notch, but they are still good, natural ingredients that are bursting with nutrition. You just have to not think 'Oh they're good for me so I'll eat my weight in them!' The reason why I am trying to hammer this point home is because once you taste something like **Katie's Beautiful Brownies** (page 265) or my decadent **Choc Orange Energy Ball Truffles** (page 257) you'll be more than tempted to have a cheeky extra. However, remember that less is more and it's all about moderation.

In this wonderful self-indulgent section, you'll find:

* **PECAN POWER GRANOLA BARS** (page 255)
* **CHOC ORANGE ENERGY BALL TRUFFLES** (page 257)
* **SUPERFOOD ICE CREAM** (page 259)
* **APPLE & BLACKBERRY CRUMBLE CRUNCH** (page 263)
* **KATIE'S BEAUTIFUL BROWNIES** (page 265)

Each and every one has been created to satisfy even the sweetest of cravings whilst making sure only good, wholesome and natural ingredients are used. Sometimes, for our own sanity, we need to go beyond the salad and if you're going to surrender to the sweet — do it right!

Remember to snap a pic of whichever sweet treat you choose to make and share it on social media to help spread the **Super *fast* Food** message and help to make a difference.

#superfastfood

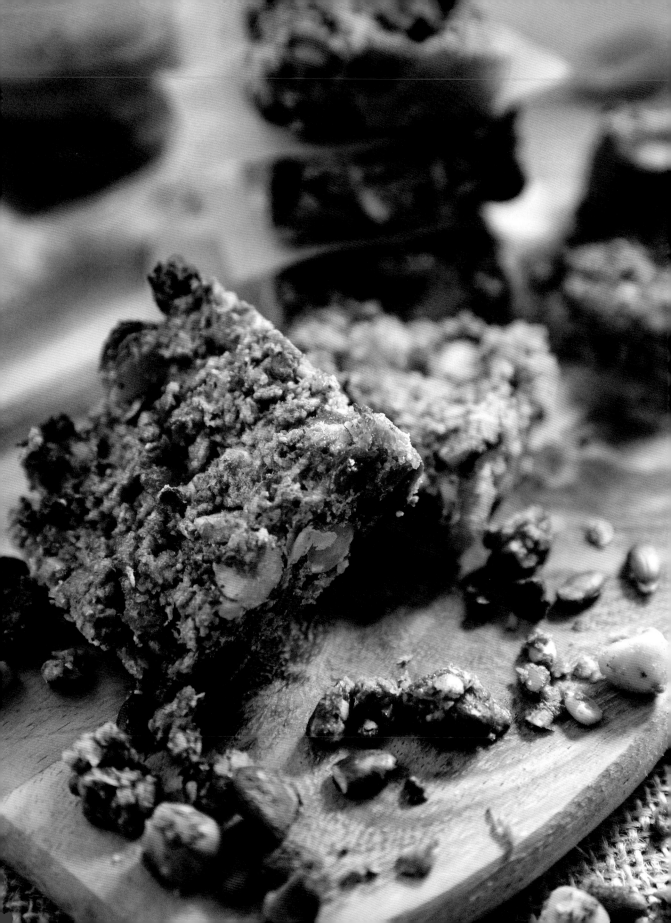

PECAN POWER GRANOLA BARS

If you've never made homemade granola bars, you are in for a real treat. What's really cool about these is not only are they super quick to make, but you can also make a large batch and store in the freezer (to keep them extra fresh) and then just eat them directly from the freezer, as they wont actually freeze! As with everything in this book, the nutrition aspect is just as important as the taste and these gorgeous bars have both in spades. Dates are rich in several vitamins, minerals and fiber. They also contain healthy oils, calcium, sulfur, iron, potassium, phosphorous, manganese, copper and magnesium. The pecans, almond butter and pumpkin seeds add some essential fats and amino acids, as well as B vitamins. Whoever said healthy can't be tasty has never tried these babies.

GLUTEN-FREE

VEGAN

VEGETARIAN

CONTAINS NUTS

INGREDIENTS:

(makes 8 - 10)

Dates (Medjool if possible)
8
Pecans
50g or 1 handful
Oats*
90g / 3oz
Cold Mineral Water
90ml / 3fl oz
Pumpkin Seeds
30g or 1 handful
Almond Butter
4 tablespoons
Raisins
80g or 2 handfuls

PREPARE:

Preheat the oven to 180 °C (350 °F/gas mark 4).

Remove the stones from the dates and any hard ends. Roughly chop the pecans. Mix the oats and water in a bowl until all the water has been absorbed, then transfer into a small baking tray along with the pecans and pumpkin seeds and distribute evenly.

TOAST:

Pop the baking tray in the oven for 10 minutes, mixing and breaking up the oats part way through to ensure they dry out.

MEANWHILE...

Place the dates and almond butter in the container of a hand blender and blend for 20 seconds until it forms a dough. Transfer the dough, toasted pecans, pumpkin seeds, oats and raisins to a mixing bowl and lightly combine using your (clean!) hands. Then transfer to the baking tray and push down firmly with the back of a spoon or your (very clean) hands.

REST:

Place in the freezer for 10 minutes, before cutting into 8-10 lovely pieces.

*Oats are technically gluten-free but unfortunately some commercial oats have been cross contaminated with wheat, barley or rye, during the harvesting, storage, milling or processing, so be a little careful here if you are particularly sensitive.

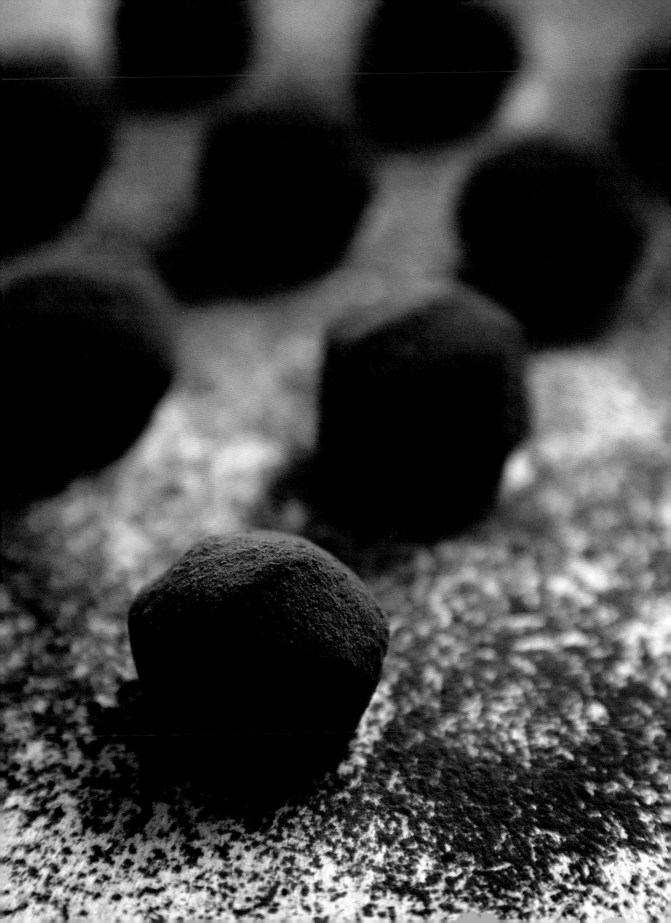

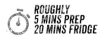

CHOC ORANGE ENERGY BALL TRUFFLES

Sometimes there aren't the words to encapsulate what you want to describe, and this is one of those times. I think on this occasion the proof of the pudding simply needs to be in the eating. You won't like me after you've tasted these, you'll LOVE me...a LOT! Although these make 10-12 balls, if there are a few of you in the household, particularly little ones, you're going to need to double or triple up on the ingredients.

GLUTEN-FREE

VEGAN

VEGETARIAN

CONTAINS NUTS

INGREDIENTS:

(makes 10 — 12 balls)

Cacao or Cocoa
15g or 2 tablespoons
Orange
1 small
Cashew Nuts
80g or 2 handfuls
Raisins
80g or 2 handfuls
Coconut Oil
1 tablespoon

PREPARE:

Spread 1 tablespoon of cacao/cocoa onto a chopping board. Grate the orange to remove the zest and squeeze the juice into a small container.

BLITZ:

Place the nuts into the container of a hand blender or *Retro Super Blend* or *Bullet* and whizz for 10 seconds. Add all the other ingredients and blend for 20 — 30 seconds.

SHAPE:

Take a heaped teaspoon of mixture, then using your (clean!) hands, shape into a ball and roll over the cocoa covered chopping board so it gets nicely coated. Repeat until you have used up all of the mixture.

REST:

Place the finished balls onto a plate and pop in the fridge for at least 20 minutes before you devour!

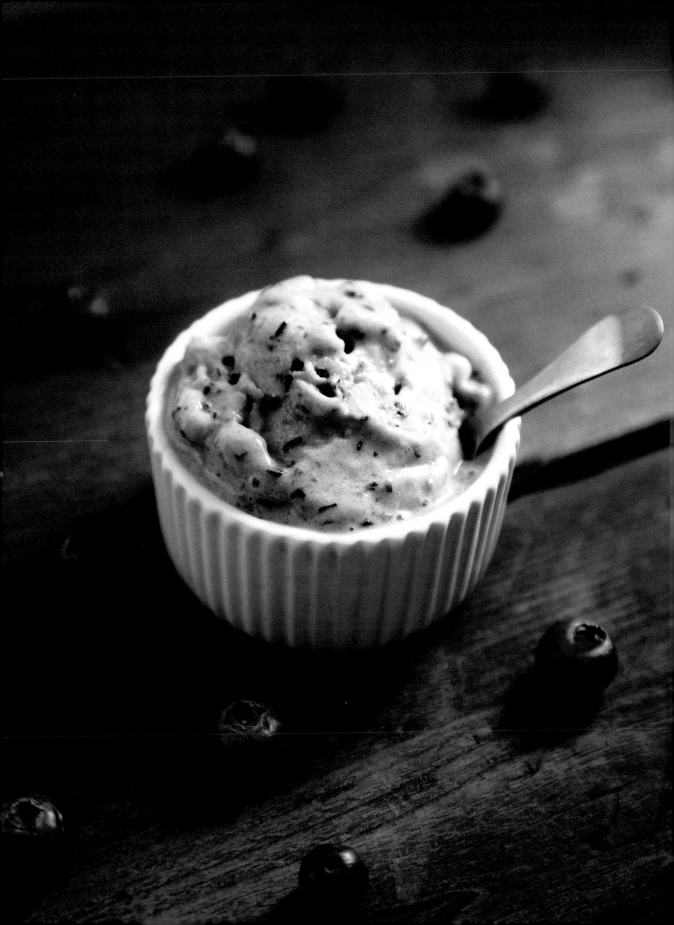

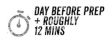

SUPERFOOD ICE CREAM

When you saw the name of this recipe I imagine you expected the appearance of either some spirulina, wheatgrass, acai or goji berries. You can of course use this simple recipe of blueberries and banana as a base and add some of those if you choose, but please don't underestimate just how 'super' these two apparently simple ingredients are. If the humble banana and blueberry were just discovered in some remote Amazonian rainforest today, they would certainly both be making headline news. I could write an entire book on the benefits of banana alone (well someone actually has!) and blueberries are the nutritional masters of the berry world. No refined sugar and it really does show those ice cream cravings where to go!

GLUTEN-FREE

VEGAN

VEGETARIAN

INGREDIENTS

(serves 2)

Bananas
2 medium
Blueberries
150g / 5oz

DAY BEFORE PREPARATION:

Peel and freeze the bananas.

MAKE:

Remove the frozen banana from the freezer and leave at room temperature for around 10 minutes. Cut each banana into 4 and place into the container of a hand blender or standard blender along with the blueberries and pulse for 30 – 60 seconds until it turns into the texture of ice cream.

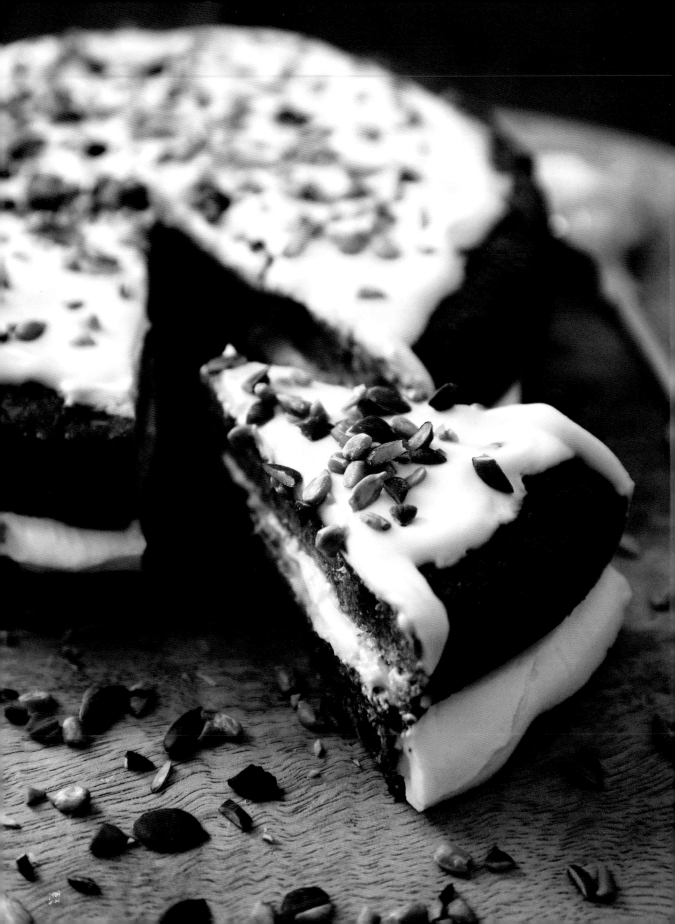

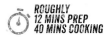

CRAZY GOOD CARROT CAKE

GLUTEN-FREE

VEGETARIAN

Carrot cake is one of my all time favourite sweets and this recipe is gluten free and contains no refined sugars or fats. Most gluten-free, healthy carrot cake recipes use two or three (or even more!) different types of flour and other unusual ingredients, but this recipe is refreshingly simple and tastes oh so good.

CAKE INGREDIENTS:

Serves – well you decide!

Carrot
2 medium

Oranges
2 medium

Eggs
4 medium (free range & organic)

Ginger
40g or 4 cm x 4 cm

Self-raising Flour (Gluten-Free)
400g or 14 oz

Baking powder
1 level teaspoon

Sultanas
100g or 4 handfuls

Cinnamon
1 heaped teaspoon

Olive Oil
200 ml or 7 fl oz

Honey
4 tablespoons

FOR THE TOPPING

Soft Cheese
250g or 9oz

Orange Juice (this will be left over from the cake ingredients)

Honey
2 tablespoons

Seeds (pumpkin or sunflower)
20g or 1 small handful

YOU WILL NEED:

2 medium, loose bottomed, cake tins.

PREPARE:

Preheat the oven to 180 °C (350 °F/gas mark 4).

Oil the inside of the cake tins and line the bottom with grease-proof paper.

Remove the hard ends from the carrots and grate. Finely grate the orange skin, cut in half and manually squeeze the juice into a small bowl. Whisk the eggs. Peel and finely grate the ginger.

CREATE:

Sift the flour and baking powder into a large bowl, then add the carrot, orange zest, grated ginger, sultanas, cinnamon and mix. In a separate bowl gently mix the eggs, oil, honey and half of the orange juice, then gradually add to the dry ingredients and mix gently. Spoon into the cake tins.

COOK:

Bake for 40 minutes. Remove from the cake tins by tipping upside down and patting the bottoms. Remove the paper and leave to cool on a wire rack.

MEANWHILE...

Place the cheese in a mixing bowl and add the remaining orange juice and honey, mix until combined and then pop in the fridge to firm up.

FINISH:

When the cake is totally cooled, spoon half the topping mixture onto the top of each cake and pop one cake on top of the other. Chop the seeds and sprinkle over the top.

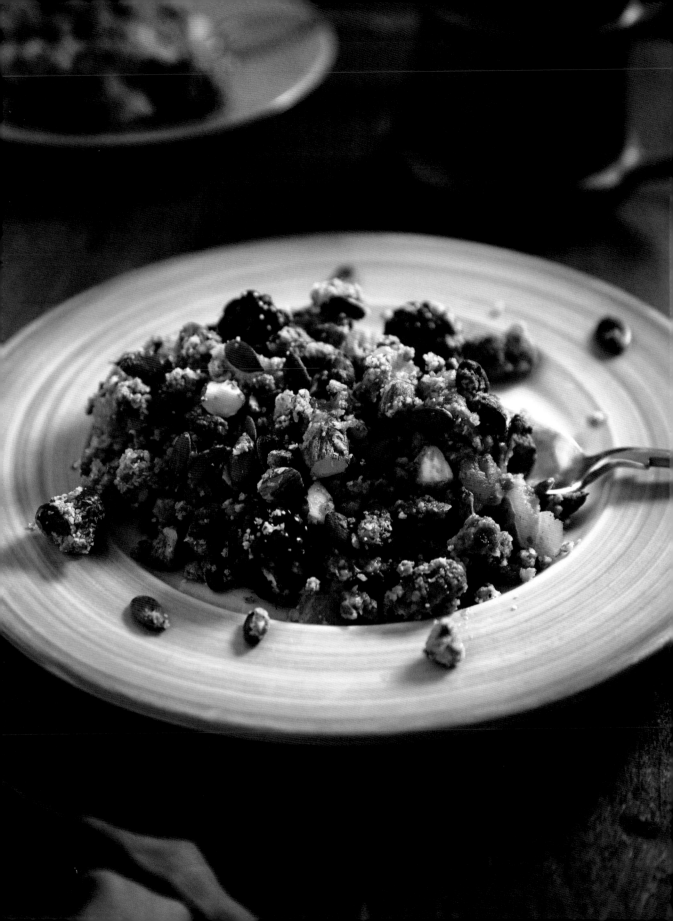

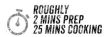

APPLE & BLACKBERRY CRUMBLE CRUNCH

The wonderful thing about this crumble is that there are NO refined sugars, NO dairy, NO wheat and NO gluten. Because there is no flour that needs cooking, it only requires 10 minutes in the oven, so it's super QUICK, super NUTRITIOUS and super FREE FROM the Big Three. Tastes wonderful on its own but a cheeky dollop of Superfood Ice Cream (page 259) doesn't go a miss either!

GLUTEN-FREE

VEGAN

VEGETARIAN

CONTAINS NUTS

INGREDIENTS:

(serves 2)

Baking Apple
1 medium

Dates (Medjool if possible)
4

Boiling Water
100ml/3.5fl oz

Blackberries
80g or 1 large handful

Oats*
60g/2oz

Almonds
30g or 1 small handful

Pecans
30g or 1 small handful

Pumpkin Seeds
25g or 1 handful

Honey**
2 heaped teaspoons

Almond Butter
2 heaped teaspoons

PREPARE:

Preheat the oven to 180 °C (350 °F/gas mark 4).

Peel the apple, remove the core, cut into small chunks and place in a pan. Remove any hard ends and the stones from the dates, chop into small pieces and add to the pan along with the boiling water.

COOK:

Place the pan on a medium heat and allow to gently cook for 10 minutes, then add the blackberries and cook for a further 5 minutes stirring occasionally.

MEANWHILE...

Place the oats, almonds and pecans into the container of a hand blender or *Bullet / Super Blend* and whizz for 10 seconds until it forms a 'flour'. Place the 'flour' into a mixing bowl along with the pumpkin seeds, honey and almond butter. Using your (clean!) hands 'crumble' the mixture.

CREATE & COOK:

Place the cooked apple and blackberries in an oven-proof dish. Sprinkle the crumble topping over the top and cook for 10 minutes.

*Oats are technically gluten-free but unfortunately some commercial oats have been cross contaminated with wheat, barley or rye, during the harvesting, storage, milling or processing, so be a little careful here if you are particularly sensitive.

** If vegan use an alternative sweetener.

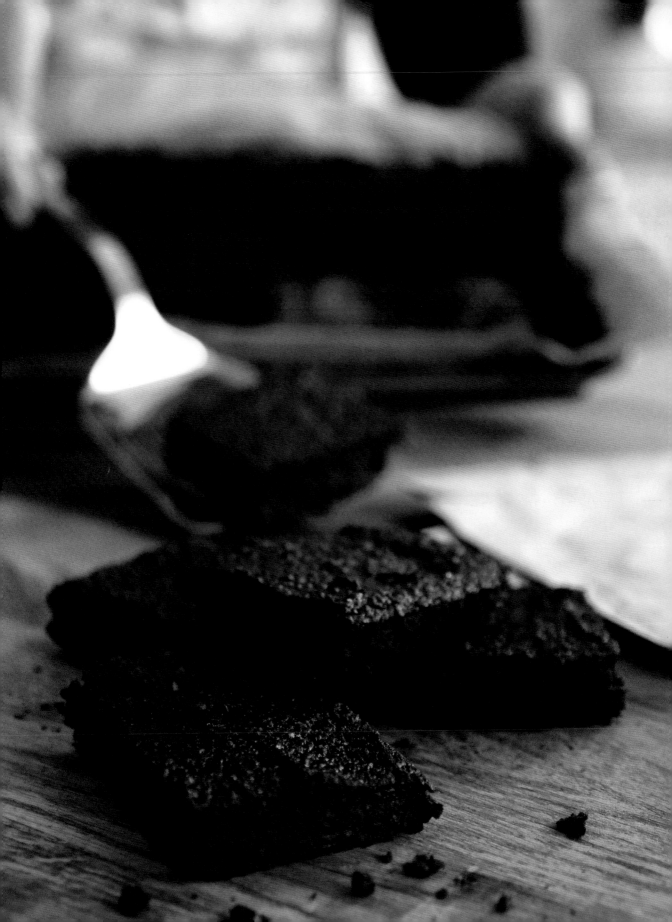

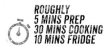

KATIE'S BEAUTIFUL BROWNIES

These are OFF THE SCALE delicious! No refined sugar, no dairy, no wheat, no rubbish! I know I am biased as Katie is my beautiful girl, but I don't do false flattery and these really are the nicest 'good for you' brownies I have ever had. It's not easy to get the balance right when using only good ingredients but Katie has nailed it. After you taste these babies you will love her almost as much as I do

GLUTEN-FREE

VEGAN

VEGETARIAN

CONTAINS NUTS

INGREDIENTS:

(makes 10 — 12 brownies)

Baking Apples
2 medium
Dates (Medjool are the best)
10 large
Almonds
150g/5oz
Honey*
3 tablespoons
Cacao or Cocoa
5 tablespoons
Boiling Water
500ml/18fl oz

PREPARE:

Preheat the oven to 180 °C (350 °F/gas mark 4).

Line a shallow baking tray with greaseproof paper.

Peel the apples, remove the cores, chop into chunks and place in a pan. Remove the stones and any hard ends from the dates.

BLITZ:

Place the almonds into a food processor and blitz for 30 — 60 seconds until they turn into almond 'flour'. Add the dates, honey and cacao/cocoa to the almond flour.

COOK:

Pour the boiling water into the pan containing the apples and place onto the hob over a medium to high heat and boil for 10 minutes. Then drain the water and add the apples to the food processor.

BLEND:

Blend the mixture for 30 — 60 seconds until all combined, then scoop the mixture into the baking tray.

COOK:

Place in the oven and cook for 20 minutes, until the top goes firm.

COOL:

Allow the brownies to cool at room temperature for 20 minutes, then place in the fridge for 10 minutes before cutting into 10 — 12 pieces.

* If vegan use an alternative sweetener.

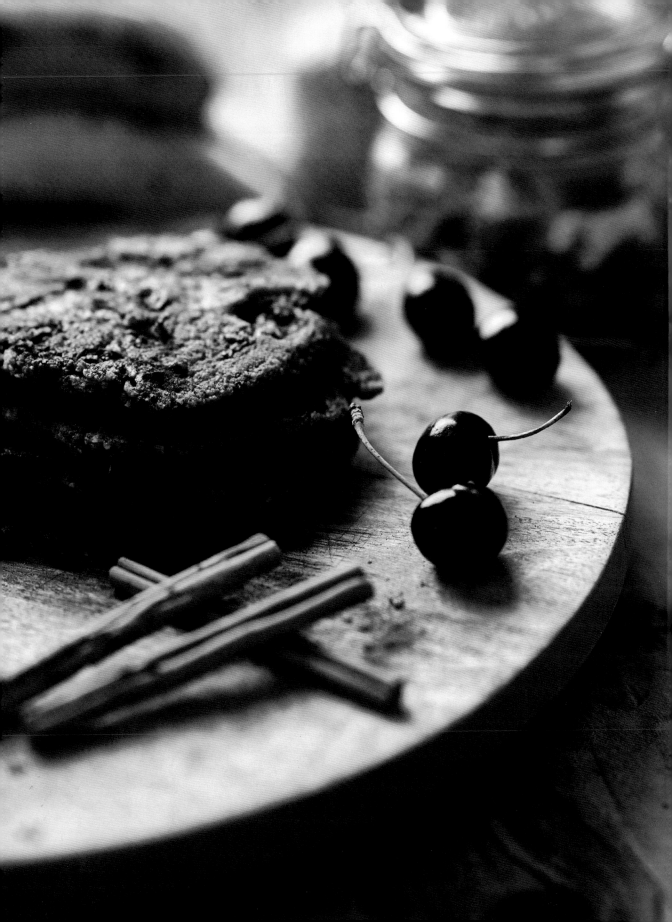

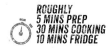

KATIE'S BEAUTIFUL BROWNIES

These are OFF THE SCALE delicious! No refined sugar, no dairy, no wheat, no rubbish! I know I am biased as Katie is my beautiful girl, but I don't do false flattery and these really are the nicest 'good for you' brownies I have ever had. It's not easy to get the balance right when using only good ingredients but Katie has nailed it. After you taste these babies you will love her almost as much as I do

GLUTEN-FREE

VEGAN

VEGETARIAN

CONTAINS NUTS

INGREDIENTS:

(makes 10 – 12 brownies)

Baking Apples
2 medium
Dates (Medjool are the best)
10 large
Almonds
150g/5oz
Honey*
3 tablespoons
Cacao or Cocoa
5 tablespoons
Boiling Water
500ml/18fl oz

PREPARE:

Preheat the oven to 180 °C (350 °F/gas mark 4).

Line a shallow baking tray with greaseproof paper.

Peel the apples, remove the cores, chop into chunks and place in a pan. Remove the stones and any hard ends from the dates.

BLITZ:

Place the almonds into a food processor and blitz for 30 – 60 seconds until they turn into almond 'flour'. Add the dates, honey and cacao/cocoa to the almond flour.

COOK:

Pour the boiling water into the pan containing the apples and place onto the hob over a medium to high heat and boil for 10 minutes. Then drain the water and add the apples to the food processor.

BLEND:

Blend the mixture for 30 – 60 seconds until all combined, then scoop the mixture into the baking tray.

COOK:

Place in the oven and cook for 20 minutes, until the top goes firm.

COOL:

Allow the brownies to cool at room temperature for 20 minutes, then place in the fridge for 10 minutes before cutting into 10 – 12 pieces.

* If vegan use an alternative sweetener.

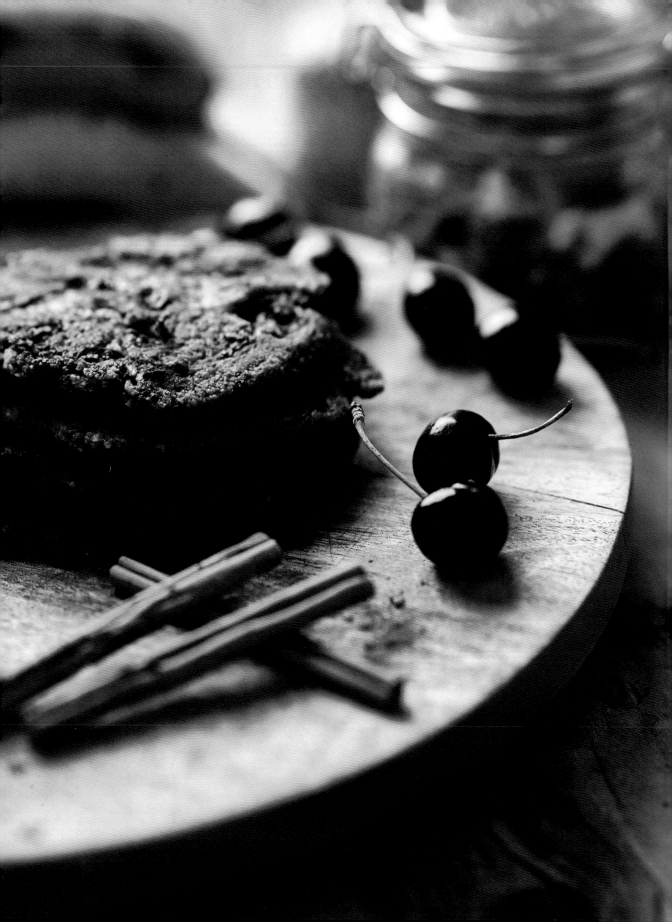

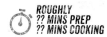
GOOEY CHERRY AND ALMOND PANCAKES

I was planning on writing a full written intro description for this recipe as I have for all the others, but two words will do the trick:

UTTERLY RIDICULOUS!

That's it and that's all — Enjoy.

GLUTEN-FREE

VEGETARIAN

CONTAINS NUTS

INGREDIENTS:

Serves 2

Cherries
8
Oats*
50g /2 oz
Almonds
75g/3 oz
Banana
½ medium
Honey **
1 heaped tablespoon
Ground Cinnamon
1 teaspoon
Filtered Water
100ml/3 fl oz
Coconut Oil
1 tablespoon

PREPARE:

Cut the cherries into quarters and remove the stalk and stone. Place the oats and almonds in a large container of a hand blender or *Retro Super Blend* and blend for 10 — 15 seconds until they form a flour.

NEXT:

Add the banana, honey, cinnamon and filtered water and blend for 10 — 20 seconds until the mixture forms a batter. Then add the cherries and mix.

COOK:

Place the coconut oil in a frying pan and heat over a medium to high heat, then add a quarter of the mixture to the pan and shape into a pancake and cook for 2 — 3 minutes each side, until golden. Repeat using the rest of the coconut oil and mixture. Depending on the size of your pan, you can probably cook two at a time.

SERVE:

Enjoy these amazing little pancakes, whilst warm and gooey.

*Oats are technically gluten-free but unfortunately some commercial oats have been cross contaminated with wheat, barley or rye, during the harvesting, storage, milling or processing, so be a little careful here if you are particularly sensitive.

** If vegan use an alternative sweetener.